More Praise for

Five Steps to Selecting the Best Alternative Medicine

"An indispensable guide to assist us through the patient/physician partnering process. It is a book that would greatly benefit all who read it."

— Benjamin Shield, coauthor of *Healers on Healing*

"A must for anyone puzzled about the varieties of alternative health care."

— Beverly Rubik, Ph.D., author of
The Interrelationship Between Mind and Matter

"This book is a shopping guide of sorts. If you follow its suggestions, you may do a better job of finding the best alternative health care provider for you."

— John E. Upledger, D.O., author of *Your Inner Physician and You*

"This book would be helpful to anyone who wants the best alternative medicine can offer."

— Mrs. Norman Cousins, author of *Caring for the Healing Heart*

"This book will make a sorely needed contribution toward demystifying the process of obtaining alternative medical care. In an age when options seem to be expanding faster than our ability to comprehend them, the Mortons' book will be a guiding light in the often dimly lit hallways of America's alternative medical care system."

— Janet F. Quinn, Ph.D., R.N., F.A.A.N.,
Associate Professor and Senior Scholar,
Center for Human Caring University of Colorado Health Sciences

"This book fills an invaluable need for those seeking help for their medical needs. It brings answers to the many questions which are currently being asked."

— Evarts G. Loomis, M.D., F.A.C.S.

Five Steps to
SELECTING
the Best
ALTERNATIVE
MEDICINE

Five Steps to SELECTING *the Best* ALTERNATIVE MEDICINE

A GUIDE TO COMPLEMENTARY & INTEGRATIVE HEALTH CARE

MARY & MICHAEL MORTON

NEW WORLD LIBRARY
NOVATO, CALIFORNIA

New World Library
14 Pamaron Way
Novato, California 94949

© 1996 Mary & Michael Morton

Editorial: Gina Misiroglu
Cover & text design: Linda Corwin
Cover photograph: Comstock

"A Doctor's Story" is reprinted with permission from Iona Marsaa Teeguarden, M.A., The Joy of Feeling: Bodymind Acupressure (Tokyo/New York: Japan Publications, 1987), p. 168.

Library of Congress Cataloging-in-Publication Data

Morton, Mary, 1957 – .
Five steps to selecting the best alternative medicine:
a guide to complementary and integrative health care /
Mary and Michael Morton;
foreword by Joan Borysenko; preface by Bernie Siegel.
p. cm.
ISBN 1-880032-94-5 (pbk. : alk. paper)
1. Alternative medicine — Popular works. 2. Consumer education.
I. Morton, Michael, 1947 – .
II. Title.
R733.M676 1996   96-36134
610 — dc20   CIP

First printing, December 1996
Printed in Canada on acid-free paper
ISBN 1-880032-94-5
Distributed to the trade by Publishers Group West
10 9 8 7 6 5 4 3 2 1

DEDICATION

Mary:

To my parents, Richard and Mary Walker and Elizabeth and George Vulich, for their support and love.

To my grandmother, Mimi Spencer, who introduced me to alternative medicine and who showed me that the best way to age is to become young at heart.

To Norman Cousins, a generous mentor and an inspiration.

To the One who leads us back to Soul.

Michael:

To my parents, James A. Morton and Joy and Douglas Edlund, who taught me the importance of compassion and forgiveness.

To my grandfather, Isaac Soskin, who believed in me when no one else could.

To my dear friend and mentor, John Earl Fetzer, who opened the world of alternative healing and medicine to me.

To the True Word and the One who embodies it, who sets us free from the need to be healed.

TABLE OF CONTENTS

FOREWORD

by

Joan Borysenko, Ph.D.

Over the years I have worked closely with hundreds of patients whose encounters with healing professionals — ranging from Western-trained doctors (allopaths) and psychotherapists to bodyworkers, acupuncturists, naturopaths, and shamans — have both helped and hindered the process of healing. I have found that no matter what tradition they come from, the healer's efficacy ultimately depends on the same key elements: suitability of their craft to the illness in question, the skill with which they practice, and their personal qualities as a human being. The more secure they are in their own worthiness, the more healers are able to tolerate the inherent uncertainty of the healing arts, honor their patients' emotions, be responsive to their own emotions, and provide what psychiatrist Avery Weisman calls "safe conduct" through any illness, even those whose physical outcome is death. It is this health care provider that *Five Steps to Selecting the Best Alternative Medicine* helps you to find for yourself.

A few years ago I experienced a physician with this healing combination first hand. I was in a serious automobile accident and I escaped unscathed, save for one small part of my anatomy.

My nose — having struck the steering wheel when my shoulder harness failed to catch — had been opened like the hood of a car and nearly ripped off my face.

After the paramedics arrived at the accident and strapped me onto a trauma board, they asked, "What hospital do you want to go to?" Fortunately I had a ready answer. In 1981 I had cofounded and subsequently directed a mind/body clinic at Boston's Beth Israel Hospital. I knew that the hospital had top-quality medical staff and — just as important — it had a "healing feeling." Soft carpets absorbed sound, pleasing colors soothed anxiety, and the entire staff really seemed to care about the patients. This was immediately evidenced by my surgeon: a "complete" healer — a doctor in the fullest sense.

When I arrived at the hospital, he calmed me with gentle words and relevant medical information; I could feel my heart-rate decreasing and my anxiety subsiding. Then, before hooking up the IV antibiotics and preparing for surgery, he asked very simply, "Do you pray?" When I said yes, we shared, as trusting partners, a moment of silence — a very important moment for me. This physician was the embodiment of a true healer: he had technical skill, appreciation of the mind/body connection, and spiritual awareness. During that very frightening situation, he helped me to bring forth wholeness from within, rather than offering treatment merely as an intervention from without.

Yet, more often than not, in the Western allopathic medical tradition, doctoring has become less and less an art and a part-nership. Impressive technological breakthroughs have promoted a model in which patients are often "done to" and dominated rather than consulted and educated. I have come to refer to this method of practicing medicine as the "dominator model."

Because the doctor I was working with was a doctor in the fullest sense, my experience of healing from this accident was rich with positive personal meaning and my recovery was quickened.

I became acutely aware of the dangers of the dominator model when my father contracted leukemia eighteen years ago.

Although the cancer specialist we chose had impeccable scientific credentials and practiced at a well-known university teaching hospital, he was authoritarian, arrogant, and took complete control of the treatment. He insisted on the aggressive use of high doses of cortisone, which helped to lower my father's white blood count but had the unfortunate effect of making my father manic, hostile, irritable, and unable to focus. As a result, during the last year of my father's life, we could hardly talk to this man who once had been so wise, gentle, loving, and caring. Mother begged the doctor to take Dad off the drug, but he refused. When the doctor was forced to discontinue the drug temporarily in order to do more surgery, Dad regained his sanity and became horrified at the prospect of losing himself to the cortisone again. Helpless and unable to find his way through the medical maze, he seized control the only way he knew how. He jumped to his death in the middle of the night from a thirty-fifth story window.

Over the last few decades public awareness has changed substantially so that the dominator model so prevalent in modern medicine and its doctor-as-God image has tarnished — just as my father's physician's image tarnished for me. Today people want more say in their treatment and less reliance on technology for technology's sake. They have become less content to put their bodies, minds, or souls in the hands of "experts" and more likely to want to know why they became ill and how they can participate in their own healing.

Moments in history when the pendulum of public awareness swings are replete with both danger and opportunity. The greatest risk in this case is that we will embrace a new theory of medical care that is diametrically opposed to — and therefore just as extreme as — the system we are attempting to reform. The theory that we are 100 percent in control of our health, for example, is as absurd as the idea that we are nothing more than passive victims of germs, with no role to play in our healing except to follow the doctor's orders. The "truth" and the most promising philosophy of health care — lies somewhere in between.

In the last fifteen years, as medical consumers have shaken

off the mantle of passivity, they have turned to a wide range of alternative models of healing, both to supplement Western medicine and sometimes to replace it. And this presents an opportunity. The potential for taking responsibility for our health and integrating the best conventional and alternative medical treatments into an effective package has never been greater.

Many alternative forms of health care are low-tech and low-cost and are often more appropriate than a standard conventional medical treatment might be. When most of us go to a doctor, for example, we are not in need of major technological miracles. Studies indicate that some 75 percent of visits to the family doctor are for stress or anxiety-related illnesses, or for ailments such as colds or flu that will usually get better on their own. Many of us go to the doctor, then, for education, emotional support, and a helping hand in mobilizing our body's own capacity to heal. We go to be heard and encouraged. And this is where we are most often disappointed, since even the most sensitive physician is severely limited by the constraints of a typical ten-minute visit.

Depending on the nature of our problem, we might be better served by a psychotherapist, a bodyworker, a course in stress management, a chiropractor, an acupuncturist, lessons in meditation or creative imagination, or even a support group. These techniques tend to rely on restoring the body's natural balance rather than overwhelming the system with powerful drugs or procedures, and are therefore less likely to create treatment-related, or iatrogenic, damage. Many alternative healing techniques also encourage taking responsibility for our overall well-being and thus promote healthier and more fulfilling lifestyles.

The danger with alternative medical treatments is that some are unresearched and may not be effective. In some cases natural remedies may even do harm. Practitioners of alternative treatments may be poorly trained or even untrained, and in places where there are no licensing requirements even the rudimentary quality control that licensing ensures is missing. One of the worst scenarios is when an alternative treatment precludes a patient from taking advantage of a standard medical procedure that has a better chance of being curative. Clearly caution is needed in evaluating and using the wide range of alternative treatments available.

Given the number of scenarios possible under the treatment of an alternative provider — M.D. or not — learning how to choose wisely for ourselves is a necessity in today's alternative medical marketplace. And the Mortons have produced a simple, responsible guide that helps you do just that.

Taking charge of your own health can take both the courage to stand up to authority and a good deal of adeptness at sorting through sometimes confusing information about the efficacy of various treatments. Understanding the choices for healing, in both conventional and alternative medicine can be a daunting task. *Five Steps to Selecting the Best Alternative Medicine* provides invaluable information that helps you sort through those many choices so that you can come to your own informed decision.

Healing is most likely to occur when effective treatment is coupled with a partnership between patient and practitioner — as with my own surgeon. This book explores with you the dynamics of the healing partnership and how to form one for your own health care.

Not all alternative care providers are able to provide that partnership. My former mother-in-law had an experience with a chiropractor that illustrates what could have been the worst combination — ineffective treatment carried out by a dominator relationship. A friend had recommended a practitioner in another state who seemed to "work wonders" using nutritional programs. My former mother-in-law consulted him by mail and then by phone for her chronic headaches and neck tension that allopathic physicians had been unable to alleviate.

Before investing hundreds of dollars to fly halfway across the country to see him, she asked my ex-husband to phone the doctor and check him out. The doctor was infuriated by the phone call. When my ex-husband challenged the propriety of making a telephone diagnosis and asked to discuss its scientific rationale, the doctor was outraged and indignant. This is obviously the kind of "doctor" to be avoided. That is why I am so pleased with the strategies outlined in this book for screening practitioners. Using these strategies you are more likely to find a healer whose craft is suitable to your illness, who has the skill to practice it completely, and the personal qualities that will support healing.

My own positive experience with a healer-doctor and my mother-in-law's and my own father's negative experiences with dominator doctors taught me many things. I now know how important it is to be informed about your options. I also know that you need to ask the right questions *before* you start treatment if you want to be assured of getting the support you need to heal. Most of all, I now know that it is up to each of us to make sure we get the quality health care we want and deserve.

Five Steps to Selecting the Best Alternative Medicine provides the information, the steps, and the questions you need to ask in order to do all this. I think it may be the most important book you'll ever buy. Not only that, it may literally save your life.

PREFACE

by

Bernie Siegel, M.D.

Five Steps to Selecting the Best Alternative Medicine is written for the survivor. It can inspire and provide valuable information coupled with a common sense strategy that encourages one to take care of oneself in an empowering way. This book will help you find all your treatment options, which is important because a treatment that may be poison for one patient can be a gift to another.

I recently spoke at a medical school graduation. I showed the graduates slides of drawings done by patients. I wanted them to see that one patient draws an operating room as a horror while another patient draws it as an incredibly beautiful place of healing. I wanted them to appreciate that the right treatment for one patient may be the wrong treatment for another.

If you don't know what your health care options are, then someone else is going to make your choices for you. That's where the trouble may start. If someone else prescribes your options for you, you will probably have far more side effects and complications. If you decide for yourself how to respond to your illness, odds are you will have fewer side effects, fewer complications, and a greater chance of surviving. With the help of this book, you can be aware of all your options and decide what is best for you.

The authors of this book also recommend that you screen and evaluate practitioners before beginning treatment. I agree. Your doctor's attitudes can be very important to you. If you feel depressed, hopeless, and helpless because of the way you are treated by your physician, it is going to depress your immune system and reduce your chances for recovery.

If you ask a health care provider questions that are important to you before you are treated, you'll know from the answers whether you will be hurt or helped by the physician's treatment and attitude. You can then avoid destructive physicians and find an optimistic, compassionate, and capable physician who will treat you properly. There is no false hope and statistics don't determine an individual's chance of survival.

Also a doctor who is your partner knows that there is more to treating a person than just treating his disease. In a partnership you don't blame each other, you work together. You're both treated like human beings. You are creating a mutual investment society.

We all want the best care we can get. If we let the "survivor" in us motivate us to do the things that will provide us the best health care options, then we will make intelligent health-care choices. Remember, all treatments are alternatives. *Five Steps to Selecting the Best Alternative Medicine* is a book about self-empowerment. It will help you make choices that will help you cure your disease and heal your life.

Five Steps to
SELECTING
t h e   B e s t
ALTERNATIVE
MEDICINE

———————

PART I

The Steps

How to Make Alternative Medicine Work for You

Medical treatments come in many shapes and sizes.

– FDA Consumer, June 1995

If you're like most people, you've probably already read or heard something about alternative medicine. It's one of the hot topics on the national news, in popular magazines, and on television talk shows. It's the subject of debate and discussion among neighbors and close friends. Not only that, this "new" health care option has brought into question many of America's accepted medical treatments and practices.

It may surprise you to know that alternative medicine is not "new." Many of the alternative medical treatments considered new have actually been practiced for millennia. For example, there is evidence of medicinal herbs being used over sixty thousand years ago by our ancestors. [1] Further, acupuncture treatments successfully used to treat certain diseases in China over three thousand years ago are the same treatments recommended by the World Health Organization (WHO) today. [2] What is "new" is the growing interest and acceptance of alternative medicine as a viable treatment option in the modern Western world.

With so much exposure, media attention, and even contro-versy, perhaps you are wondering if alternative medicine is right for you. Possibly, you're not really sure what alternative medicine is, or even how to find the alternative medical treatment(s) that might work for you. If this is true for you, then information that gives you a working knowledge of alternative medicine is what you need. With this information, you can gain both the confi-dence and skills to determine if alternative medicine is right for you, and if it is, to move in this new and unfamiliar world with confidence.

Most likely there is an alternative medical treatment that exists to meet your current health care needs. The chances are also very good that there is an alternative health care profession-al you'll want to work with. More important, a step-by-step process exists that will help you choose, in an informed and intelligent manner, the right alternative treatment and the best alternative health care professional for you and your family's health care needs. You'll find this process and other valuable information in the chapters ahead.

This book is designed to provide you with a roadmap to make your journey into the terrain of alternative medicine a clearly defined and well-chosen one.

Mary's Story: Persistance, the Right Treatment, and a Good Partner Can Create a Miracle

"I'm sorry, Mary. There is nothing that can be done for your condition."

The year was 1972 and I was six-teen years old. Sitting in the doctor's office, I had been eager to hear how he would fix the nagging pain in my upper back. I came for solutions and support. I received neither.

I sat stunned and silent. The doc-tor proclaimed that I had scoliosis, a condition in which the ver-tebrae of the spine rotate upon each other and the rib cage becomes deformed. He said I had a severe case and proceeded to describe the bleak future he was certain would soon be mine. I would lose all sensation in my toes and fingers. My menstrual cycles would grow increasingly painful and childbirth would be complicated, at best. The pains and spasms in my back would drastically increase. The twists and turns in my spine would contort even more in the coming years, wreaking havoc on my body. There was nothing anyone could do to stop it. He said the pain I felt now was just the beginning; there was more to come.

As I struggled to absorb his prognosis, each new horrible symptom he uttered felt like a physical blow. I was determined to maintain my composure, for this doctor's bedside manner was as cold and icy as his prognosis. He offered no comfort in his voice or his eyes. I was not about to admit my immense need for reassurance in the confines of his office, even though I desperately felt it.

Finally, he finished his endless list of horrors and prophesy of doom by ordering me to withdraw from all the physical activities I loved most — volleyball, basketball, running, and dance. In his opinion, the stress from these sports would speed up the inevitable onslaught of complications. Yet he gloomily predicted that stopping my activities would only postpone the inevitable degeneration.

My mind reeled from his verdict of a future I refused to accept. I was frantic to regain some semblance of hope for my future. "Doctor," I said, "I know that you say that you can't help me with this condition, but there must be someone who can." He looked at me with eyes of steel. "There is nothing *anyone* can do."

In an instant, it seemed my life had changed completely and irrevocably. I had arrived at his office considering myself a normal, basically healthy teenager with back pain. Now I was confronted with a new and frightening view of myself and my future.

I staggered out of his office with the words echoing in my head that I had a permanent spinal disorder that would deny me the life I loved. I didn't want to accept what I heard. I felt as if a thief had stolen the rich variety of life choices I believed were mine and I wanted them back!

I walked block after block in a daze, overwhelmed by frustration and fear. Finally, after several hours, I came to the conclusion that the only way I could move forward in my life, to feel some semblance of control of my future, was to make a critical choice.

I could either accept his grim prognosis, or I could prove him wrong and create for myself the bright future I had envisioned.

I had heard of people who had defied the absolute authority of doctors' diagnoses. My grandmother Mimi had exhibited courage in the face of tragic news when, many years before, an eminent doctor had proclaimed she would only live to forty-five. I remember when she was eighty-five she was more vibrantly alive than most people twenty years younger. At ninety-two she passed on, having lived a rich, extraordinary life. My grandmother achieved this remarkable feat by searching for and doing anything that would help her heal. She was both a model and an inspiration for me.

As I remembered others' remarkable health successes, I felt an anger rise from deep inside me. I don't want to just accept this prognosis, I thought. Doctors aren't gods, and they can't know everything. Maybe there is a cure that this particular doctor doesn't know about. Maybe a cure will be found in the future. Anything is possible.

I made my choice. I decided not to accept his sentence of ever-failing health. With that decision, I experienced an inner certainty that someone, somewhere would help me heal my back. I was going to find that person no matter what any doctor said. It was here I began my long journey back to health.

After my prognosis, I started a series of consultations with various conventional M.D.'s. Some suggested a surgical procedure riddled with dangerous risks to straighten my spine. Other doctors suggested a body cast to prevent my spine from curving further. The side effects of this procedure were unpleasant, to say the least. I couldn't agree to either of these medical treatments despite the growing numbness I noticed in my toes. It was at this point I decided to explore treatments outside of mainstream medicine.

I tried a variety of alternative treatments and techniques as the years crept on. Chiropractors' spinal manipulation techniques helped relieve some discomfort, but not one of the many chiropractors I saw offered me any permanent solution for my scoliosis. Acupuncture also helped relieve the muscle tension related to my spinal curves, but the relief, again, was temporary. One friend referred me to a woman who used naturopathic treatments. She was helpful with digestion complications associated with scoliosis; however, her techniques offered no long-term solutions to my nagging back problem.

At that point I hit a wall. I couldn't find any other techniques or treatments to try. I talked to all the health care providers I knew — conventional and alternative. No one had a solution or a suggestion I felt I could agree to. So I decided to keep my eyes and ears open — and hope.

As the years went by and the dreaded symptoms increased, I feared I would never find the way to heal my back. But seven years after my initial diagnosis, a miracle happened. I finally came upon an alternative health care technique that could offer me a lasting solution.

At the time, I worked with a company that produced personal-growth workshops. It was there that I made an important new friend. Tom was open and friendly; and in our beginning conversations we found that we had a lot in common — philosophies of life, goals, hobbies, even mutual friends. One day he noticed I was in some physical pain. He asked me about it and I shared with him some of the details of my back problem. He said, "I used to have that. A pretty serious case of it too. I got rid of it through deep tissue bodywork." Bodywork! I'd never heard of such a thing! Elated, I prodded him for every detail he knew about bodywork and how it had worked for him.

The type of bodywork that had helped Tom heal his scoliosis was a special form of deep tissue bodywork called *Hellerwork*. He explained to me that deep tissue bodywork focuses on changing the structure of the muscles and the soft tissue in the body. By using deep pressure and friction, it is possible to change the actual shape of the body, much as you might change the shape and form of a soft clay doll.

Hellerwork was developed by Joseph Heller in 1979 and involves a combination of deep touch, movement education, and verbal dialogue. It focuses on both structurally realigning the body, and on facilitating an awareness of the mind/body relationship through interactions between client and practitioner. In addition, some sessions of Hellerwork focus on movement education where the client learns how to sit, stand, lift, and walk in a way that supports the unique design of his or her muscular structure.

In deep tissue bodywork, the actual position and shape of muscles are changed by using direct pressure with fingers and/or elbows to make short "strokes" on fascia (fibrous layers covering muscles). Through these strokes, muscles are molded, almost like sausages, and are either lengthened or shortened depending on what shape is needed to hold skeletal structure (bones) in correct balance. Sometimes through molding the muscles in this way, the positions of bones can be moved. Deep tissue had changed the positions of Tom's vertebrae so that his spine now "hung" straight.

Now I felt some hope again — finally. I was eager to find a practitioner of bodywork to work with me. However, later that same day — before I even began that search — I received an invaluable gift.

Eric Andresen was a practitioner of Hellerwork, and he had participated in a personal-growth workshop I had facilitated. During the workshop, he had gained many important insights and wanted to thank me for my contribution by offering me a gift of eleven sessions of his bodywork. I was flabbergasted. Knowing now what potential Hellerwork might hold for me, I enthusiastically accepted.

At our initial meeting, Eric greeted me warmly and asked about my health and what I wanted to accomplish during the bodywork sessions. I shared with him the details of my condition and my hopes for healing my curved spine. While he listened, he nodded his head in understanding. My case made sense to him. He couldn't guarantee that he could reverse all of the curvatures, but he thought he could help.

He then showed me the massage table and the room where we would work. Charts and pictures of human anatomy decorated his walls. It was pleasantly lit and I felt I could be comfortable there. Next, Eric explained what I could expect during the sessions. He said that I had an important job during our sessions together: to manage my mind. He said that lasting results were more likely if I visualized my tight muscles relaxing when he put pressure on what he called "trigger points." If I wanted an improvement in my condition, I would have to actively participate in the treatment.

Soon after our meeting, I called Hellerwork's association and verified that Eric had completed his training and was certified. Knowing that made me more comfortable about agreeing to his treatment. Intuitively, I liked this professional. His training and his technique checked out. So I decided to trust this man and I began treatment.

He began our first session with confidence. His self-assurance helped to calm my anxiousness. The more I began to feel comfortable, the more we operated in sync with one another. When he gradually applied pressure, at first barely noticeable, I started to feel a painful protest from my tightened muscle. I imagined the muscle as a sponge, offering no resistance to his pressure. It wasn't an easy exercise. I had some false starts. Then, just as the image became clear — real to me — the muscle relaxed, the pain became unnoticeable, and Eric was able to make the necessary change to the muscle.

Over time, our sessions evolved almost into a dance, rhythmic in its give and take. I filled my lungs to capacity, then began to exhale, holding in my mind an image of my muscle accepting the coming pressure. Only then did he slide his finger to the knotted muscle and gradually pressed, just enough. Intuitively he knew my limits. Eventually I coaxed him to add more pressure because I noticed that the more he used, the more headway we made.

After completing the eleven sessions, we surveyed our progress. Together we looked at my reflection in the mirror. Then we compared my "before" and "after" photographs. Neither of us spoke for a while. I didn't know what to say. The curve so prominent in my back in the "before" photographs was barely noticeable in the "after" photographs. My right shoulder, once twisted forward, was evenly balanced with my left. My knees no longer bowled in. Looking at my reflection, I saw more improvement than I ever thought possible. The body that now stood in front of the mirror looked like it was somebody else's.

Eric said he'd never seen anything like it before. I only knew that I couldn't have done this with just any person. Just when I was thinking that it was Eric's commitment, skill, and compassion that helped to create our success, he turned to me and said he couldn't have done it without me.

It has been sixteen years since my sessions with Eric and I'm grateful to say that the results of those sessions have, for the most part, held. But besides the elation I felt about reversing the growing numbness and physical discomfort that scoliosis created, this experience became a model for me of what the "best" of alternative health care is and what it can be for anyone.

In the years since working with Eric, I never forgot the value of persistence in finding a solution to my condition. I also remembered the confidence in knowing that the health care provider I was working with was competent and well trained. In addition, I had an invaluable experience of *partnering* with a health care professional. I am certain that it was our partnership that tipped the scales toward a full recovery of my previously "unhealable" condition.

The Ten Most Commonly Asked Questions About Alternative Medicine

An ever-increasing amount of information about alternative medicine is entering mainstream media. Even with all that is being written or said about alternative medicine, many people feel they are not getting the facts they need to make some very basic decisions; they feel they still need to obtain some simple answers to some very important questions.

Because of this lack of knowledge or a trepidation they feel toward unknown terrain, many people are hesitant to explore the field of alternative medicine. For this reason, it is important to answer some basic questions. Below you will find the ten most commonly asked questions about alternative medicine and our answers. These answers will provide you with details about alternative medicine to help you as you begin your journey.

1. What is "Alternative Medicine"?

Because alternative medicine is many things to many people, there is no one-line answer that would define the term simply and clearly to satisfy everyone. This reason alone is why it can be so difficult for some people to get a clear sense of what alternative medicine is — and what it is not. The truth is that one simple definition can't possibly describe all that is now considered "alternative medicine." Given this, what follows are several "answers" to the question, all considered to be "right" according to various experts.

Alternative medicine is made up of a rich array of techniques, modalities, and medical systems that are, for the most part, still unfamiliar to the majority of the public. They are, therefore, as a whole, an "alternative" to what most Americans are using when they need health care.

Much of what is labeled alternative medicine comes to us from other cultures or from ancient healing traditions. For example, the use of herbs as medicine is an ancient practice found all over the world. Acupuncture comes specifically from ancient China and has been documented as being in use as early as 2697 B.C. [3]

Interestingly, some of what is labeled alternative medicine originated in the United States. Chiropractic medicine, naturopathic medicine (as a formal system of medicine), and osteopathic medicine all have their origins in the U.S.

Contrary to popular belief, many alternative medical techniques are used everyday by people from all walks of life. *Prevention* magazine's *New Choices in Natural Healing* explains, "While the term *alternative medicine* may conjure up some pretty exotic images, many of these therapies are more familiar than you think. If you've ever massaged your temples to ease a headache, applied an ice pack to a sprained ankle, or listened to your car radio to de-stress during a traffic jam, you've already practiced some simple natural healing techniques." [4] So whether you were aware of it or not, it is likely you have already used alternative medical techniques in your own life.

In fact, the World Health Organization estimates that between 65 and 80 percent of the world's population (about 3 billion people) rely on traditional (read: "alternative") medicine as their primary form of health care. [5] They further state that when these traditional medical treatments are introduced into Western culture, they are seen as complementary or alternative.

Many of the techniques and treatments in the domain of alternative medicine are also "packaged" under a number of other labels today. The more popular of these are unconventional medicine, holistic medicine, complementary medicine, integrative medicine, integral medicine, preventative medicine, and environmental medicine.

"Alternative medicine" is also defined by what it is not. According to David M. Eisenberg, M.D., of Harvard Medical School, alternative medicines are "medical interventions not taught widely at U.S. medical schools or generally available at U.S. hospitals." [6] Wayne Jonas, M.D., director of the Office of Alternative Medicine (OAM) at the National Institutes of Health

(NIH) gave the OAM's definition: "Complementary and alternative medicine is defined through a social process as those practices that do not form a part of the dominant system for managing health and disease." [7] These two definitions, though currently accurate, will soon be dated. An increasing number of medical schools are now offering courses in alternative medicine for their students, and some hospitals already have alternative medicine departments.

The term alternative medicine can also be considered as a *code word* for a whole series of significant changes and challenges occurring within the American health care system today, including:

- The realization, that, contrary to previously held beliefs, conventional biomedicine (the medicine that most people are familiar with: antibiotics, surgery, chemotherapy, etc.) cannot solve all of America's health problems
- The growing acceptance that health is more than just "the absence of disease" and involves more than just the physical body
- The growing body of scientific research, as well as public awareness, that many alternative medical treatments are more effective, more economical, and less invasive and less harmful than conventional medical treatments
- The growing number of informed health care consumers who are open to trying alternative medical treatments and demanding to be treated as a person — not as a diagnosis — by their health care providers

As stated earlier, each of the above "answers" is considered to be the "right" answer by various groups of experts on the subject. Possibly each of these experts has a part of the answer and not the whole answer. If that is so, each is worthy of consideration when seeking a definition of just exactly what "alternative medicine" is — and is not.

2. What is the difference between alternative medicine and conventional medicine?

Generally speaking, most high quality alternative medicine is founded on six core principles and practices that differ from the principles and historical practices of conventional medicine. They are:

1. The healing power of nature first, and technique and technology second

Probably the most important difference is that alternative medicine is founded on a deep belief in the healing power of nature (*vis medicatrix naturrae*). Alternative medical providers accept that within us is a natural ability to heal, an inherent recuperative power that is the key to all healing. The alternative practitioner believes his or her job is to support and stimulate this natural healing ability inherent in each patient.

Biomedicine or conventional medicine has historically tried to reduce the healing process to a series of physiological, physical, and chemical reactions that can be measured and documented by modern science. While there is some truth in this perspective, science has proven it to be an incomplete picture of the healing process. Conventional medicine has come to place more value on the techniques and the technology rather than on the inherent healing power of nature we possess as human beings.

Conventional medicine has historically tried to replace the body's natural healing response by quickly removing symptoms. For example, instead of stimulating and strengthening the immune system to fight an ear infection in a toddler, a biomedical doctor will usually prescribe an antibiotic. The child often receives immediate relief, but at what price? The antibiotic wreaks havoc on their developing digestive system by destroying valuable "friendly" bacteria needed for good digestion. Also, the child's immune system is not any stronger to ward off the next ear infection, thus creating a dependency on antibiotics. The price of immediate relief is the threat of future long-term health problems for the toddler.

The alternative medical practitioner, on the other hand, would suggest a less drastic treatment that stimulates the body's natural healing power. Relief might come through warmed drops of mullein garlic ear oil. Immune stimulation might come through a combination herbal tincture. In truth, a full healing response could take ten days, but the long-term benefits to the child are a stronger immune system and an uncompromised digestive system.

2. Patient centered rather than physician centered

Biomedicine has historically been perceived as more "physician centered," in which the doctor's opinions and beliefs are considered more important than the patient's. High quality alternative medicine, on the other hand, is first and foremost "patient centered," in which the feelings, beliefs, and the opinions of the patient are essential elements in the treatment decision-making process.

High quality alternative medicine is founded on a deep appreciation of the wonder and mystery of being a unique human being. According to the Burton Goldberg Group's *Alternative Medicine: The Definitive Guide*, "The return to health...is a road which each person must walk according to his or her unique individuality. It is also a road that needs to address one's entire being, taking into account one's mental, emotional, and physical aspects, as well as the structural, biochemical, and energetic components that shape each of us."[8]

Conventional medicine has come to see the patient as his or her diagnosis rather than as an individual. Further, the role of the patient is a more passive one, being subjected to the authority and expertise of the doctor. Also, in the biomedical model, historically it is assumed that the doctor's skills and best judgment are the final authority. The idea of a shared decision-making process regarding treatment between the doctor and the client/patient is contrary to the traditional role that doctors have historically played in our medical system.

The origins and repercussions of this biomedical doctor/patient model is explained by author Norman Cousins:

> For the past fifty years, the practice of medicine has been dominated by the need to identify diseases and

germs. Through the discoveries made by the microscope and the advent of antibiotics, medicine became very specific and technical. This tended to make doctors mechanistic. It tended to obscure recognition of the human soul and its role in contributing to both illness and recovery. Modern medicine tended to place undue emphasis on the prescription pad over bedside manner. This emphasis on medicine and medical machinery created a critical psychological separation between patient and physician. There is no bigger problem in medicine today because when a patient has an illness, nothing is more important than the doctor's reassurance. [9]

It was the ancient Greek physician, Hippocrates, who said, "It is more important to know what sort of person has a disease than to know what sort of disease a person has." Like Hippocrates, most alternative practitioners view their clients as human beings rather than a diagnosis. This is one of the reasons that alternative medicine has become so popular.

3. Do no harm

Many alternative medical systems are rooted in the "least dramatic means" principle. The essence of this principle is, "Always use the least drastic harmful therapies first." This means that alternative medical providers, in general, choose techniques and therapies which are the least invasive or harmful to get the desired result.

In today's press, many stories have been published charging that quite often medical doctors do, in fact, harm their patients in the process of treating them. The charges range from unnecessary cesarean sections during childbirth to heart bypass surgeries which could have been avoided through diet and exercise changes. One reason for unnecessary invasive treatments is that the majority of medical doctors are not familiar with effective, less invasive alternative treatments. Historically, doctors have not been taught these procedures in medical school and many don't take alternative therapies seriously — despite the growing body of research around the world that demonstrates their efficacy.

In addition, conventional medicine has come to place greater value on the removing symptoms as quickly as possible — even if additional physical problems are created in the process. Many times a conventional treatment will bring an immediate "cure" by removing the symptoms of an illness while never addressing the true cause so that real "healing" can occur. One might say that it pulls weeds out by their tops while rarely getting to their roots.

That is not to say conventional medicine does not have a place in health care. Conventional medical interventions such as surgery, chemotherapy, radiation, and antibiotics can be real blessings in their ability to stop, slow, and, at times, heal horrible illnesses. Such medicines are important weapons in the arsenal to fight illness and disease. But alternative practitioners believe these forms of intervention should not be the medicine of first choice, given the devastating side effects that can erode a person's quality of life. They should be the medicine of last resort. However, such treatments have been the medicine of first choice for conventional doctors for years.

In their book, *Take Care of Yourself*, James F. Fries, M.D., and Donald M. Vickery, M.D., state: "Drugs interact with other drugs, causing hazardous chemical reactions. They have direct toxic reactions on the stomach lining and elsewhere in the body. They cause allergic rashes and shock. They are foreign chemicals and have severe side effects.... Under some circumstances, they probably cause cancer." [10] Though many conventional doctors would agree with this statement, they continue to practice medicine that in many cases is not really founded on the edict of "do no harm." As a result, approximately forty-five thousand patients die each year in hospitals *as a result of the conventional medical treatment they received.* [11]

In contrast, an alternative health care provider such as a naturopathic doctor (N.D.), would use a whole array of "less drastic" treatments *first* in order to help the patient to heal (unless, of course, the patient was in a life-threatening condition). The N.D. refers his or her patient to a conventional doctor for more drastic treatments only after finding that all the appropriate alternative treatments at his or her disposal could not heal the patient's condition.

4. Results generally take longer

One primary goal of alternative medicine is to stimulate the body's natural healing response and to let nature take its course. From this process, a true healing can occur, increasing the chances that the symptoms will not return. Some people find the slower rate of recovery frustrating if they are accustomed to immediate results from conventional medical treatments.

Here's an example of how this slower healing can occur: At four months, our daughter Deana had a severe case of eczema — front and back, head to toe. She was miserable. Her pediatrician prescribed a lotion that contained cortisone. We knew some of the strong side effects of cortisone (including compromised vision) and decided not to put that drug on her young skin, even though her doctor was certain it would make her eczema disappear. Instead, we decided to seek a naturopathic doctor's recommendations and made an appointment to see Rena Bloom, a licensed naturopathic physician we knew was well trained and had a special interest in infants and children.

After examining Deana and asking us many questions, Dr. Bloom suggested that Deana might be allergic to her formula. The formula she was taking was advertised as hypoallergenic for colicky babies — which Deana was. However, this hypoallergenic formula was fifty-two percent corn product, a common allergen in adults as well as children. Dr. Bloom gave us a recipe for a goat milk formula and suggested we try it on Deana. We felt very comfortable giving our daughter this formula because we had learned that goat milk's nutrient makeup is very close to human mother's milk.

After two weeks of an exclusive diet of goat milk formula, we noticed some improvement in our daughter's condition. But because we assumed that Deana's eczema should have cleared by then, we called Dr. Bloom to report our results. Dr. Bloom reminded us that she thought Deana would take a full four to six weeks to recover from the toxicity of her previous formula. She explained that Deana's system was clearing out the toxins as quickly as possible and she needed the time to heal herself. In other words, we needed to be patient.

It took Deana the full six weeks to recover. When she did, she was noticeably more alert and happy. Not only that, her skin and complexion returned to "peaches and cream."

5. Use of natural and whole substances

Many alternative treatments use natural substances such as herbs, botanicals, homeopathics, nutritional supplements, and whole foods. There is a general belief among naturopathic doctors that the use of whole or natural products to treat maladies adds more to the healing process than their synthesized counterparts. While many synthesized pharmaceuticals may be more potent and fast-acting, they also often come with unpleasant side effects.

According to John R. Lee, M.D., coauthor of *What Your Doctor May Not Tell You About Menopause*, "Most over-the-counter and almost all prescribed drug treatments merely mask symptoms.... Drugs almost never deal with the reasons why these problems exist, while they frequently create new health problems as side effects of their activities."[12] On the other hand, natural substances are believed to produce fewer side effects, though they may take longer to work. The American public appears to be aware of this. In 1993, consumers spent approximately $1.5 billion on herbal remedies.[13] As a result, more and more drugstores and shopping store chains now stock a full line of herbal supplements for their patrons.

6. Higher standard of health

For many years, health was seen as "the absence of disease" by conventional medical doctors. The common philosophy was:

If you are not sick and you do not need to go to the doctor's office or the hospital, then you must be healthy. In years past, people would go to their conventional doctors for an annual check up and be given a clean bill of health. An individual's health was assessed by the results of the physical examination. Little, if any, consideration was given to lifestyle factors such as diet, exercise, or personal or psychological issues. Minimal concern was generally given to the emotional, mental, spiritual, and social aspects of the person.

In contrast, alternative medical systems have long been founded on the premise that health is a dynamic process that most consider more than just the absence of illness. Other factors ranging from the strength of a person's "vital energy" to how happy the person is in his or her personal and professional life are also considered. The "whole person" is evaluated when determining one's state of health and well-being. In most alternative systems of healing, a person's physical, emotional, mental, and psychosocial health, his or her diet and lifestyle, as well as the person's religious and spiritual concerns are all carefully addressed when assessing health and well-being.

Fortunately, with the advent of the holistic health movement over the last two decades, a growing number of conventional doctors are now recognizing that health is more than the absence of disease.

3. My friends and family are skeptical about the merits of alternative medicine. How do I help them feel confident in my decision to use alternative medicine?

To many people, alternative medicine is still suspect. Some of this is warranted. Not all of what is labeled alternative medicine can be assumed to be good medicine. So the concern and skepticism of your friends and family is only natural. The problem is that most people who are skeptical of alternative medicine base their caution on outdated information, facts that are only partially true, or complete misconceptions. Of course, there are those who would never even consider that alternative medicine has merit, regardless of what the facts are. ("Don't confuse me with facts, my mind is made up!")

Let's look at the roots of the bias against alternative medicine: A great deal of this distrust can be traced directly to the beliefs and opinions of the conventional medical community. Since conventional medicine enjoyed an unquestioned confidence from the public for almost five decades, the public accepted the critical views about any treatments not part of conventional biomedicine. As a result, in time conventional medicine's beliefs became the public's beliefs.

According to the "Chantilly Report" to the NIH on alternative medicine, one conclusion the public reached regarding conventional medicine is that it is the "one true medical profession." This originated through the "long-standing belief held by many conventional medical practitioners that they should be the only one representative voice for the whole of medicine." [14]

Another result is the public now places an unrealistically high level of confidence in conventional medicine's high-tech diagnostic and therapeutic procedures. Many presume that if procedures are "high-tech," they must be very effective. However, evidence points to the opposite conclusion: High-tech is *not* always effective.

A case in point: A young woman checked into a major New York hospital to treat a tumor on her chest. The hospital had a new experimental group and was researching the effects of microwave hypothermia on cancer. The woman was one of the first participants in their research group. Unfortunately, the researchers didn't have adequate thermal control and miscalculated the amount of hypothermia they gave this young woman. Within moments they had burned a hole right through her sternum. She also had burns from her chin down her entire neck and halfway down her trunk. After she recovered, she exclaimed that with such high technology in a major hospital in a large city, she had been very optimistic that she would be cured. She realized, however, that she should have been less optimistic, asked more questions, and been more cautious.

In contrast, many alternative treatments are not "high-tech" and are actually seen as "low-tech." Consequently they are *perceived* to be ineffective when they actually *are* effective. For example, our neighbor's one-and-a-half-year-old son Alex had a very high fever a few weeks ago. His parents took him to a pediatrician (M.D.) for a diagnosis. When they asked about using herbs to treat his infection, his doctor's response was, "Herbs are for salads. He needs something more sophisticated to help him recover. Drugs." This doctor was convinced of this fact despite the tremendous body of scientific research that indicates that herbs could, in fact, help the boy recover. Based on the recommendations they received from a naturopathic physician about other infections that Alex had in the past, his parents decided to use herbs before trying drugs. Within twenty-four hours of administering the recommended herbs to Alex, his fever disappeared and he was markedly better.

The public has grown to prefer the "safety of the status quo," which, in the United States, *is* conventional doctors and their medicines. Because doctors routinely prescribe drugs such as antibiotics and sedatives, the public generally believes that they are the most effective treatments. However, several major magazines and national news programs have reported the hazardous side effects of these drugs. As a result, an increasing number of patients now voice their concerns about these drugs and ask about alternatives.

The most fervent critics of alternative medicine charge that alternative medical practitioners are "quacks." The NIH's "Chantilly Report" defends the alternative medical practitioner saying, "The term 'quack' generally means one who pretends to have medical knowledge but does not; that is, it implies the element of fraud. . . . [However] most alternative healers do possess some other sort of knowledge [than M.D.'s] that they and their clients believe is relevant to health." [15]

Another charge is that alternative medical practitioners prey on the gullible and uneducated. The "Chantilly Report" also refutes this, stating that, "Recent studies of cancer patients indicate that well-educated persons with higher incomes are more likely to use alternative treatments, primarily because they want to take charge of their health." [16]

When using alternative medicine, you will probably encounter skeptics with these or other misconceptions. When this happens, the best strategy is to present an "unbeliever" with real facts backed by respected sources. Generally this is a much more effective approach than sharing personal stories about miraculous cures. Irrefutable facts have a way of calming skeptics' doubts — and sometimes — of changing their minds. Here are some facts that will alleviate the concerns and doubts of the people in your life:

- Worldwide, only ten to thirty percent of people use conventional medicine, 70 to 90 percent use alternative medicine. [17]
- Approximately $22 million of U.S. government money has already been spent on alternative medical research since 1992 at the National Institutes of Health and Public Health Services. [18]
- The American Medical Association (AMA), in Resolution #514, "is encouraging its members to become better informed regarding alternative (complementary) medicine and to participate in appropriate studies of it." [19]
- Renowned hospitals, such as Columbia-Presbyterian Medical Center in New York, have created alternative medical clinics in their facilities.
- Almost one-third of American medical schools — among them Harvard, Yale, Johns Hopkins, and Georgetown Universities — now offer coursework in alternative methods. (See reference section for a complete list.) [20]
- Many alternative approaches have been scientifically proven to be less invasive, less dangerous, more effective, and more economical than conventional medicine.
- Mutual of Omaha says it saves about $6.50 for every dollar it spends covering nonstandard (read: alternative) treatments. [21]
- Seventy-four percent of the American population desire a more natural approach to health care. [22]
- Of the one out of three Americans who have used alternative

medicine, 84 percent said they would use it again. [23]

- Traditional Chinese medicine has been chosen by the World Health Organization for worldwide propagation to meet the health care needs of the twenty-first century. [24]
- The U.S. Government sponsors the use of acupuncture in drug rehabilitation programs. [25]
- There are five homeopathic hospitals in Great Britain run by the British National Service. [26]
- One out of three drugs prescribed in Germany is an herb. [27]
- One out of every ten Americans is under the care of a chiropractor. [28]
- In 1993, Americans spent an estimated $1.5 billion on herbal remedies — ten times more than was spent on over-the-counter sleeping pills from grocery stores and drugstores. [29]
- In 1991 Americans made more visits to unconventional health care providers (425 million) than to conventional doctors (388 million). [30]
- One out of three Americans were using unconventional medicine in that same year. [31]
- Americans spent almost $13.7 billion on unconventional care in that twelve-month period. [32]
- Seventy-five percent of that money was out of pocket. [33]
- Twelve percent of Fortune 500 companies offer alternative medicine as part of their health care compensation packages. That number is expected to increase to eighteen percent by the end of 1996. [34]

Despite all the facts and statistics you can offer others, when you are sure that you want to try alternative medicine, the most important information that you can offer the people who care about you is:

- You have investigated your options.
- You are confident in your choice.
- You look forward to sharing your success stories with them.

4. If I suspect there is something wrong with me physically, should I go to a medical doctor (M.D./D.O.) or to an alternative practitioner?

Most health care professionals, be they alternative practitioners or medical doctors, recommend that you first go to a conventional medical doctor or to an osteopathic physician to get a diagnosis. D.O.'s and M.D.'s receive extensive training in diagnosing pathology (illnesses and diseases). If you visit an alternative medical practitioner who has not had the vast experience and training in diagnosing pathology that a conventional medical doctor or osteopathic doctor has, that person might miss a problem that could mean your very survival. Dr. Len Wisneski, corporate medical director for Marriott Corporation, says, "Many times a patient will come to me after they have been working with an acupuncturist. I have found problems that the acupuncturist missed. If we are looking at cancer, there is some precious time that has been lost, which we could have used to combat the malignancy." [35]

After you have had a thorough examination, a diagnosis, and a recommended treatment program from an M.D. or D.O. then look at alternative medicine for other treatment options that might be as effective and less invasive. Of course, if you are in a crisis situation where time is of the essence, you will need to determine if you have the luxury of time to find an alternative. In a critical situation, your first and foremost commitment is to stay alive. In that case, conventional medicine may be your best answer. If this is not the case, we encourage you to look at all your alternative options.

Also, we encourage you to find a conventional doctor who will work with you as a team player as you explore your alternatives. Dr. Joe Jacobs, former director of the Office of Alternative Medicine at the National Institutes of Health says, "Keep your medical doctor informed about any alternative therapies you are trying or want to try. If you feel he or she is biased against alternative medicine, find another medical doctor. But maintain a relationship with an M.D [or D.O]."[36] Just because there are shortcomings in our conventional medical system, don't underestimate the tremendous skills, training, and value a medical doctor can bring to your health care. A conventional medical doctor or an osteopathic physician is an important part of your health care team.

The biomedical system is usually your best source for getting a fast and accurate diagnosis. Always use conventional or osteopathic medicine first if you suspect you have a potentially life-threatening health problem.

5. There are so many different kinds of alternative medicine. How do I know that I'm choosing the right kind?

It can be overwhelming to realize just how many alternative techniques and treatments are available today. The answer is to learn how to find the appropriate alternative medical options for you in an easy, efficient manner. The information presented in Step One of this book will show you how to do that. It clearly explains how to find the most effective treatments from around the world for your health condition. It also can get you to information on how to "live well" while living with your health condition, thus enhancing your quality of life. By doing Step One: Learn your Options, you will gain the information and knowledge you need to make informed and wise decisions about which alternative treatment is right for you.

To further support you in this, we have provided a list of relevant organizations, support and advocacy groups, computer search services, and Internet research sources in the Reference Section of this book.

6. I've heard there are some charlatans in alternative medicine. How do I know who is well trained and competent and who is not?

In conventional medicine, there are both good and bad practitioners. The same is true for alternative medicine. For this reason, it is important to educate yourself. Steps One through Five of this book are designed to give you the tools you need to get the right information about *any* modality of alternative medicine so that you are not swayed by blind faith, by faulty information, or "a good line."

Also, in Part II of the book, you'll learn what is considered competent training for the five licensed general health care providers of alternative medicine: the M.D. as an alternative medical practitioner, the Chinese medical practitioner, the chiropractor, the osteopath, and the naturopathic physician. This will help you discriminate effectively in choosing any of these alternative practitioners.

You, as well as every health consumer, have both the right and the responsibility to make educated decisions about who should treat you and how. This book is structured to give you the tools you need to determine how well the alternative health care provider is trained, if he or she is fairly priced, and if he or she is able to give you the health results you seek.

7. Is alternative medicine safe?

This is another question that does not have a simple answer. In this country, "safe" means a treatment method has been endorsed by the Food and Drug Administration (FDA). Most of the treatments that are labeled as alternative medicine have not yet received this endorsement, and it's possible they never will.

In the "Chantilly Report" on alternative medicine, it states that "the current Federal mechanisms of regulating medical research do not favor the evaluation of many forms of alternative treatment. Because the costs of developing, evaluating, and marketing new drugs are so prohibitive, pharmaceutical companies are not likely to invest time and effort in therapies, such as nutritional or behavioral approaches, that cannot be patented and are therefore unlikely to offer the opportunity to recover their investment and provide a return to stockholders. This means that many alternative therapies are likely to be casualties of the formal research process." [37]

This information indicates that health care consumers need

to look beyond the recommendations of the FDA when making health care decisions — especially when one considers that other countries have regulatory systems, similar in function to the FDA, that have competently evaluated the effectiveness of many alternative therapies. Europe, for example, takes note of substances that have a long history of effective use and approves them under "the doctrine of reasonable certainty." This rule parallels the World Health Organization's (WHO) Guidelines for the Assessment of Herbal Medicines, which states that a substance's historical use is a valid way to document safety and efficacy in the absence of scientific evidence to the contrary.

European and the WHO assessments of alternative remedies are available to you. You will need to personally decide whether or not the World Health Organization and Europe's standards of safety are adequate for you. While you ponder the issue, consider the following: In comparison with the rest of the world, the United States ranks fifteenth in life expectancy — behind Japan, Iceland, Sweden, Switzerland, Hong Kong, the Netherlands, Norway, Canada, Spain, Australia, France, Cyprus, Greece, and Italy. Further, the United States is ranked number one among the industrialized nations of the world in infant mortality, death of children under the age of five, AIDS, cancer among men, incidences of breast cancer, and malpractice lawsuits. [38]

You can reasonably assume that licensed alternative providers use treatments and techniques that are safe when used correctly. If you have a question about a particular treatment or remedy recommended by an alternative health care practitioner, ask both that practitioner and other experts to provide you with as much information as necessary to determine if you can personally have confidence in the recommended treatment.

8. Will my insurance cover alternative medicine?

The answer to this question depends on the state you live in and your insurance company. For example, many states now have a law that requires all health insurance policies to cover licensed chiropractic doctors. So, if you are in one of those states, you are legally entitled to receive chiropractic care and be reimbursed by your health insurance according to the terms of your policy. Your treatment must be defined as "medically necessary" and, at most insurance companies, conventional medical doctors decide if a licensed chiropractic doctor should be treating you or not. In the language of the trade, the conventional doctor is the "gate-keeper" who decides which procedures warrant reimbursement.

What does this mean? Because many M.D.'s do not appreciate the viability and effectiveness of the chiropractic paradigm, the process of determining "medical necessity" is usually biased against many chiropractic medical claims. Conventional doctors decide that such treatment is not "medically necessary" in many cases. There are even documented cases of insurance companies stating that they will pay for expensive pain-relieving drugs or surgery from an orthopedic surgeon rather than pay for a much less expensive series of chiropractic adjustments to treat the same problem. Some insurance companies have made this choice even though competent research has shown the chiropractic approach to be an effective treatment for the same condition.

Still, there is hope, as ever-increasing numbers of insurance companies are taking a serious look at the importance of covering alternative medical treatments in their health policies. Mutual of Omaha now covers chiropractic, Prudential pays for acupuncture, and Blue Cross of Washington and Alaska offers a plan entitled "AlternaPath," which covers licensed naturopathic doctors. Also, a growing number of hospitals and HMOs are including alternative medical services in the treatments provided for their patient-customers.

Prevention magazine's *New Choices in Natural Healing* says the most comprehensive insurance plan covering alternative medicine today is American Western Life Insurance Company of Foster City, California. Ayurveda, homeopathy, nutritional counseling, massage, and physical therapy are all covered in their Wellness plan. The company includes a full-time Wellness

Line with naturopathic doctors "on call" for their customers.

The Wellness plan costs 20 percent less than their traditional plans, because, says Wolf Klain, president of American Life, "We believe very strongly that if people do take care of themselves, if they take preventative measures, it's only going to save us all a lot of money in the long run." [39]

We suggest contacting your health insurance representative to get the facts on possible reimbursement for alternative medical treatments. If it turns out that your plan is "biased" against reimbursement for alternative medical treatments, we encourage you to shop around and find a plan that is better suited for your health needs.

Insurance plans covering alternative medicine are growing at a surprising speed. One successful HMO, Oxford Health Plans, is over one million members strong in the New York Metropolitan area. They surprised the industry by heavily committing themselves to covering preventive medicine using alternative medical techniques. Although their alternative medical plan is still in development, other HMOs are watching to see if this commitment will eventually turn into profits for Oxford. If so, we can only anticipate that more HMOs will follow in Oxford's footsteps. [40]

Also, if you live in Washington state, you are in luck. Washington now requires that all health insurance companies cover all licensed and certified alternative practitioners. Although Washington is the only state in the union to pass such a law, it is possible that other states will follow suit. [41]

9. Will alternative medicine work for me?

No system of medicine can guarantee success for every condition. Each system of medicine has certain health conditions for which it is best suited and some health conditions for which it would be the treatment of last choice. This is true for conventional medicine as well as alternative medicine.

An example is Chinese medicine, which has a long and respected history of treating conditions of infertility and impotence in less drastic and more natural ways than conventional medicine. Many couples who were unable to conceive have become happy parents after receiving a series of treatments of Chinese herbs and acupuncture for their condition.

The key to success with alternative medicine is to make sure you have all the accurate information you need from around the world about treating your health conditions. It can also get you information on how to "live well" while living with your health condition, thus embracing life. By doing Step One as outlined in this book, you can be assured of finding the right alternative medical treatment for your health care needs if one exists. Becoming familiar with good research from throughout the world on your alternative medical choices increases your chances of getting the results you want.

10. Is there a way for me to responsibly seek out good alternative medical care for myself and my family?

The five steps described in the upcoming chapters is the best answer to this question. By participating in Steps One to Five, you *can* responsibly and wisely choose good alternative medical care for yourself and your family. Whether you are just beginning your exploration of alternative medicine or you have been using alternative medicine for some time, following these five steps will allow you to make good decisions about *any* modality of medicine. And incidentally, in most cases, by following the five steps, you can save time and money, too.

The Five Steps are:

Step One: Learn Your Options — Add to your M.D.'s recommendations by researching the latest resources to get all your treatment options.

Step Two: Get Good Referrals — Find referrals through various sources and verify that these referrals have the capability to really help you.

Step Three: Screen the Candidates — Make use of an alternative practitioner's staff to get reliable information about the provider and how they work.

Step Four: Interview the Provider — Ask the provider *all* the pertinent questions to know if you can confidently work with this professional.

Step Five: Form a Partnership — Maximize your healing potential by developing an active alliance with your alternative health care provider.

Each of these steps — and how to do them competently — are outlined in the next five chapters of this book. When used together, they form a process that will lead you through the maze of alternative medicine to the results you desire.

There is one important point to consider in order to use this book to your best advantage. For all of us, our relationship to our own health is an ever-changing process. Health care needs alter as we mature and grow and live life. As a result, these five steps, as well as the chapters in Part II, will be useful to you in different ways as your needs change in their focus and intensity.

For instance, if you are in a health emergency, diagnosed with a life-threatening or debilitating disease, your motivation for gathering *all* the relevant information and finding just the right health care provider will be significant. You will want to be thorough in both gathering and evaluating information because you won't want to miss anything important — like the key to your relief and/or remission.

In a serious health care crisis, doing each detail of all five steps in this book will serve you well because each step is designed to be as complete as possible. Each step is presented so that you see "both sides of the coin" — so that you don't miss any important details, thus compromising your ability to get the health results you really need.

On the other hand, if you have a minor health care complaint, such as a digestive problem that is at the very worst annoying, you probably won't need to complete all of the recommendations in each of the five steps. You might not have the motivation, the need, or the time to check every information resource regarding digestion, gather a full list of referrals, and ask every pertinent question of the staff and the provider.

However, if a friend had great success with relieving her digestive complaints through an N.D., and you would like to try this provider but really don't know much about naturopathic doctors, parts of this book will be helpful to you. The chapter on naturopathic doctors will familiarize you with the naturopathic philosophy of medicine, typical treatments used by N.D.'s, what happens on a first visit, and N.D. associations and professional groups. After skimming through Steps One through Five you might get some ideas about how to partner with this provider. Perhaps you'd like to check that the N.D. graduated from an accredited college. Verification that this provider is qualified, along with other details you learn about N.D.'s, will help you feel more comfortable on your initial office visit, as well as assist you in making the most of your time with this health care professional.

Whatever your particular needs when using this book, we encourage you to use it in the way that is best for you. It is not necessary to do every suggestion in this book for every health care need you'll have. Pick and choose. Do what *you* need to do to get the health care results *you* want.

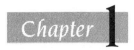

STEP ONE: LEARN YOUR OPTIONS

Becoming an Informed Health Care Consumer

One of the nicest things in life is to have a mission. And to know that it's supported by a great deal of valid information can only strengthen one's confidence in that mission.

– Norman Cousins[1]

Knowledge is power. Whether you are looking for information to enhance your health or searching for the answer to reverse a terminal illness, you'll want all the credible information you can find about your condition. And rightly so, because gathering all the reliable information you need to make informed choices about your health condition not only gets you the treatment that can remedy or enhance your health care situation, it also empowers you.

By learning your options in Step One, you can take greater control of the type and quality of health care you receive. By working with your primary health care provider and the other six key information sources outlined in this chapter, you can find all the information you need to make informed and intelligent health care decisions for yourself. By learning your options, you become a savvy health care consumer, no longer bound to one doctor's opinion or one medical system's answer to your health care needs.

Michael's Story: Seven More Years for Dad

In 1986 my father was in excruciating pain. After visiting a cancer specialist, he was told that he was suffering from a relapse of prostate cancer, which had metastasized to the bones in his legs and back. After his doctor told him he had less than six months to live, he gave up all hope.

Another doctor had treated him with radiation ten years before, when he was first diagnosed with prostate cancer. But now, since they told him that further treatments might help the pain but would not prolong his life, he refused to receive any more radiation. "They've burnt me enough! No more!" I remember him saying.

At that time, I began working for the Fetzer Foundation, whose mission was to support scientific research of alternative medicine. My work at Fetzer brought me into the very center of the alternative health care arena and, eventually, to the key to my father's very survival.

At the Fetzer Foundation, I was privileged to work for one of the most phenomenal men I have ever met, John Earl Fetzer. John Fetzer was a millionaire many times over. At one point he was one of the five hundred richest people in the United States. Of all the areas in life he could choose to spend his money, he chose to fund the new frontiers in science and medicine that honored a holistic perspective of the human being.

During my first week on the job, John Fetzer gave me the assignment of "getting the big picture" in alternative medicine and healing. He said, "We need to get the lay of the land before we fund any further research. Go to it!" I was to determine what was worth funding among all alternative medical practitioners, projects, and programs from around the world. I was to go wherever I needed to go and to meet whomever I needed to meet in order to complete this assignment. Needless to say, this began one of the most amazing journeys of my life.

I traveled the world and met some extraordinary people and experienced fascinating cultures with impressive alternative medical treatments. I met with the Dalai Lama in India and discussed how Tibetan Medicine could benefit AIDS patients. I met with Shamans from South America and witnessed them diagnosing and treating illnesses in people on the other side of the world. As a result of such meetings, I came to appreciate how medical systems from ancient cultures could help heal the illnesses of our own modern world.

In my meetings with rare and gifted healers who made tumors disappear in a matter of minutes, I was challenged to accept that not all that is real and possible can be explained by science.

I also met quacks and charlatans who I saw take money from terminally ill patients by playing on their fears and hopes. Because of such people I learned very quickly that we all need to keep both of our eyes open while we open our minds to learn about the new and unconventional.

My work also took me to Senate hearings that debated certifying alternative medical education as well as research committee meetings that examined the role of prayer in the healing process. The questions and concerns raised in these meetings made me realize that many people are suspect and even fearful of alternative medicine simply because it is unfamiliar and challenges the status quo.

One particular meeting in which I participated provided me with information that helped add precious years to my father's life, which cancer and his doctor would have stolen from him. The focus of the meeting was to review the results of a research project the Fetzer Foundation had funded. The project documented and catalogued case histories of spontaneous remission from terminal illnesses with little or no medical intervention. ("Spontaneous remission" is when all the symptoms associated with an illness disappear.) The sources for this material were credible and respected scientific medical literature from around the world. The draft research document that was reviewed in that meeting catalogued *hundreds* of documented spontaneous remission cases.

Fortunately, because of my position, I was able to share this research about spontaneous remission with my father seven years before it was made public. I asked him to read my copy of the draft document as a favor to me. He did. And the data from that report moved him so much that from that day forward he became inspired to find new hope for healing and living.

During my time at Fetzer, I also learned that there were other treatment options for my father's cancer that were unknown to his doctor. Together, my father and I began to search for the answer his cancer doctor said did not exist.

It was through a patient advocacy group called Patient Advocates for Advanced Cancer Treatments, Inc. (PAACT) that we found a treatment that was being used in Europe and Canada but was not available or even legal in the United States at that time. It was a new drug called "flutamide." We managed to get the drug sent to us from a doctor I knew in Canada. Soon after starting this drug, my father's pain went away. Better still, his cancer went into remission, adding another seven good years to his life — that not only benefited him, but myself and many others as well.

Some years after his remission, I was visiting him at his home in Texas. Out of the blue he said, "Thank you!" Puzzled, I responded, "What for?"

"You saved my life," he said. "First of all, you gave me that book on spontaneous remission that showed me that I didn't have to die. And second, you helped me to see that there were other options for my medical care than what my doctor told me. If it was not for these two things, I would have been dead seven years ago. You gave me the time I needed to make peace with myself and God and to do some more good in this world. Thanks, son."

"I'm just glad you're still here, Dad," is all I could say as tears streamed down my face.

This experience with my father taught me a great lesson. Although a conventional drug saved him, *never* will I blindly accept a doctor's treatment recommendations — especially when a doctor says that "the condition is terminal." I know now that there are many effective treatments that most M.D.'s are just not aware of. More importantly, I am certain that if there is a treatment that will help a physical problem of mine or a member of my family, I *will* find it.

WHAT YOU WILL LEARN IN THIS CHAPTER:
* *How to empower yourself in your healing process*
* *The seven key sources to good health care information*
* *The three-question test for complete and dependable health care information*

How to Empower Yourself in Your Healing Process

Historically, in the Western conventional health care system, the doctor has been the leader; the patient has been the follower. What the doctor said, the patient gratefully accepted. When the doctor decided on a treatment, the patient consented. To question the doctor or to even suggest another option was taboo. In fact, getting a second opinion has become an accepted practice only in the last fifteen years. Today, almost all of this is changing; in fact, not getting a second opinion for most health issues is practically unheard of.

Now, health care consumers from all walks of life are demanding a more active role in their health care. And they are right to make that demand because science has found that patients who play a more active role in their health care actually stimulate their immune systems, which helps their bodies heal. You can take advantage of this immune enhancement yourself by becoming an alert participant in your health care instead of a passive observer.

Taking back your power in the doctor/patient relationship probably sounds like a good idea, but is not always easy to do. The fact is most of us have grown used to relinquishing power and responsibility to the doctor. Most of us consider the doctor to be the "expert" who knows what is "best" and whose job it is to "fix" us. As long as we continue to hold these beliefs, it may be difficult for us to balance this historically one-sided relationship and to empower ourselves.

To become empowered in any area of life, we must be willing to take responsibility for our part in the decision-making process. To be responsible, we need to be "able to respond." Learning about our health condition and our options enables us to respond with competent, informed choices.

Here is some information to consider as you begin to be more actively involved in your own healing process:

1. Health care providers can't be experts on everything.

Many people wonder why a well-trained M.D. who diagnoses a condition wouldn't know all the relevant treatments for that condition. After all, the doctors are the experts, aren't they? Isn't knowing all the effective options the doctor's job? Yes, it is supposed to be. But the fact is that new information about health care treatment options is exploding to such a degree that no physician could possibly keep up with all the recent scholarship and research. More importantly, very few conventionally trained M.D.'s are familiar with the alternative options that might be available for your condition.

Bernie Siegel, M.D., well-known surgeon and author of *How to Live Between Office Visits* (HarperCollins, 1993), agrees and says that the average doctor would have to spend *two* to *four* hours a day on research alone just to stay abreast of the latest advances. [2]

Add to this the fact that different doctors have different opinions about the best treatment for a particular condition, and you soon realize that you may not get the best information available on which to base your decisions.

Some people may find this shocking — especially if they have never questioned their doctor's authority. But consumers who want all the relevant information about treatments for their condition have to take charge and get it themselves. One cannot assume that a doctor knows about all the credible treatment options.

2. If your health care professional doesn't like you being informed, you need to find a health care professional who welcomes your input and desires to contribute to your recovery.

Jan Guthrie found that her doctor didn't appreciate her research. In the early 1980s, she was diagnosed with a rare type of ovarian cancer called granulosa cell tumor. The suggested treatment after her emergency surgery: radiation therapy. Jan found herself in shock when first given this information.

In an effort to regain control of her life, Jan started research to find all the information she could about her condition and what she could do to offset any negative side effects. Through her research, she discovered that radiation therapy did not keep granulosa patients alive any longer than those who opted for regular checkups after surgery.

When she shared her findings with her oncologist, he discounted her research and efforts to be informed about her cancer. Fortunately, Guthrie did not cower at the doctor's response and began a search to find a doctor she could work with, who respected her efforts to empower herself.

Guthrie did what all health care consumers must do if they come across a health care provider who is intimidated by their patients' research: fire that professional and find another. Guthrie did just that. Through additional research, she found a doctor who had a successful track record in treating granulosa. Not only that, he was someone she felt she could talk with and be heard.

After a series of surgeries, she is now in remission. Further, as a result of her experience, Jan has founded one of the best medical information services available, The Health Resource. Details on this information service are described later in this chapter.

3. Good health care professionals welcome informed patients.

Actually, many excellent health care providers are relieved when patients come to them informed about their condition and treatments. In some ways, it takes the pressure off them. Dr. Christiane Northrup, past co-president of the American Holistic Medical Association and founder of the Women to Women clinic in Yarmouth, Maine, is a good example of a health care provider who enjoys working with informed patients. She says, "I love it when my patients come in with articles and books. I get a sense of what they know and where they are starting. If they have two or three different opinions on how to handle their condition, then I'm off the hook in a way. I don't have to be God. I can immediately step off my pedestal and be a partner." [3]

Dr. Northrup is among a growing number of conventional medical doctors who support their patients in becoming informed and educated participants in their own healing.

4. Gather as much information as you can, but don't believe everything you read or hear.

Substantiate and cross-check any information you believe might help your health condition. In a state of enthusiasm, it can be easy to veer off into an unproductive or even dangerous direction. You don't want to waste valuable time and money with treatments that divert you from getting the results you really want. More importantly, it can put your life or health at risk. Check to be sure that the "new" information is going to support your long-term health goals.

Joan Borysenko, Ph.D., author, medical scientist, and psychologist, shares an example of a patient of hers who took the wrong advice to heart. "I had a patient who had read one of the many books over-promoting the theory of illness-as-metaphor. She came in with a sore, stiff shoulder, convinced that her problem was caused by her inability to reach out and take what she wanted in life. My lifelong experience as a woman, however, quickly led me to a different diagnosis — one that I had previously applied to myself. Eyeing her purse, which looked like a feedbag for a stallion and easily weighed as much, I decided that a better metaphor for her shoulder was pack-rat-ism. When she lightened her purse, her shoulder pain disappeared." [4]

Remember that not all information is fact. By cross-checking all the information you find about your condition, you protect yourself from potential harm and from inappropriate, as well as potentially dangerous, treatments.

5. Becoming informed takes some work.

Research requires more effort than relying on the expertise of health care professionals. Again, if you want results, you increase your chances of getting those results, if you are in charge of getting the facts.

Lon Nungesser, a long-term survivor of AIDS, is an inspiring example of the miracles you can create by taking charge of your health care. He was diagnosed with an AIDS-related terminal cancer in 1983. Although his doctors gave him three to six months to live, he did not give up. He was angry that at thirty years of age he was facing imminent death. "I held on to that anger and used it to mobilize myself to gather information," he says. "I went to medical libraries and read everything I could about the disease. Even if it took me some time to understand the information, I didn't care. The information process was powerful and informative. It is probably eighty percent of the reason I went into remission." [5] Through his research, Lon Nungesser developed his own treatment program that put the AIDS into remission for eleven life-filled years — ten more years than the doctors predicted.

Getting informed will take some time and energy on your part, but the benefits and rewards will far surpass the effort involved.

6. Medical terminology can be difficult to understand.

If you are not trained in the medical profession, the terminology can be difficult to understand. But don't let that hold you back. Remember, they're only words. And with some effort, you can learn what those words mean.

Realize that the time you invest to understand the information you find in medical journals, you read in pamphlets, and you hear during a doctor's visit, will always pay off, primarily because understanding your condition as well as all the viable treatments is empowering. And that can significantly help you to reach the health results you desire.

If you are intimidated by technical information, you can get some help. Here are some suggestions:

- Speak with friends or associates in the medical profession who can help you understand medical terminology.
- Consult medical dictionaries, which are available in libraries and bookstores. They'll help you make sense of what you are reading. If they are too intimidating, there are many good scholarly journals, such as the *New England Journal of Medicine* and *Alternative Therapies in Health and Medicine*, that can also help you understand current research and terminology. Finally, "lay journals," such as *Prevention*, *Natural Health*, and *Townsend Letter*, offer support in some technical language.
- Find information services that offer glossaries of terms in the information kits they send you about your condition. Their glossaries are clearly written and designed for the layperson.

Use the diagnosis you get from your doctor as an opportunity to get more information. It might take some work, but you'll be empowered by both the learning process and by what you learn.

The Seven Key Sources to Good Health Care Information

There are seven major sources to good health care information that can assist you in finding all your treatment options. They are sources that anyone can use. Some of them are sources of information that most physicians do not conventionally use. Many times, using these sources can give you the latest information about your health condition, which your own physician may not know.

The seven key sources to good health care information are:
1. Your doctor and other health care providers
2. Other patients and their friends
3. Libraries
4. The Internet
5. Medical and health information service organizations
6. Advocacy organizations and support groups
7. Professional organizations and trade associations

1. Your doctor and other health care providers

In spite of the shortcomings of conventional biomedicine, in most cases there is no finer system of medicine for gaining an accurate diagnosis of your health condition. The technological advances and the diagnostic tests available to you in conventional medicine are in a class of their own. Blood and urine screenings can check for everything from the presence of cancer to vitamin and mineral deficiencies, from pregnancy to cardiac risk. Sonograms that show birth defects in an unborn infant, and MRIs that can detect the smallest of brain tumors, help make conventional medicine the first choice when seeking an accurate diagnosis. So, first and foremost, see your doctor for the best chance of a fast and accurate diagnosis for most health conditions.

Getting a diagnosis from an M.D. or D.O. is particularly important if your health condition is life-threatening. If you suspect that this might be the case, you will want to get an accurate diagnosis as quickly as possible. Be wise — always use conventional doctors as one of your sources for getting a competent diagnosis for your condition.

In conjunction with using a conventional medical doctor, make use of any other health care providers who are familiar with you as a patient. Don't feel you have to depend on just one type of doctor or health care provider when getting a diagnosis. The insights that a health care provider trained in another medical system might have into your physical condition could be useful in your search for solutions to your health needs. In fact, some diagnostic techniques of alternative medical systems can detect subtle imbalances that conventional diagnostic techniques can miss.

2. Other patients and their friends

Mary's story in the beginning of this book is a great example of how productive this information source can be. After years of "keeping her eyes and ears open," it was her new friend Tom who shared with her a technique that was, at the time, unfamiliar to her, but had greatly helped him heal the same condition she suffered from: scoliosis.

Seek out, through your own network of friends and health care providers, other individuals who have healed themselves of the health condition with which you are diagnosed. Keep in mind that a treatment which worked for others may or may not work for you. However, if you can find three people who healed themselves with the same treatment, you may have found a treatment option with great potential for *you*.

Once you have a treatment option you think might really help, explore the details of how this treatment works, who is trained to offer the treatment, and its success rate by using the other six key sources to good health care information.

3. Libraries

Within a few miles of your home, you have access to one of the greatest resources of information in the world for your health care needs, the public library. Today, we truly have a "system" of libraries, many of which are interconnected by computers that offer you a health information resource of Goliath proportions.

There are two types of library systems available to the public. They are your local community and county libraries, and university and medical school libraries.

Your local community and county library system: Local libraries are either part of a municipal or a county library system.

Most of these in the U.S. are also members of a state library system, which is usually connected to the Library of Congress and the National Library of Medicine by way of the Internet.

University and medical school libraries: University libraries can be a direct resource of in-depth information about most health conditions. In many cases, research reports, critical analysis, as well as other important information about your health conditions can be easily found or accessed.

To make the most of either type of library, your best friend is the Reference Librarian. Not all libraries use the same information storage products or search services. Therefore, it is important to first check with the reference desk to learn what information options are available at the library you are using.

Most libraries offer the following services which can assist you in learning your health care options:

The periodical index: Through this library service, you can access any articles that have been written in the popular press (i.e., magazines, journals, and newspapers) about your health condition. Some libraries even offer a specialized periodic index that focuses on health-related issues. This special index not only lists the published articles and health-related pamphlets, but also can bring up the actual text for you to either review or print.

On-Line Public Access Catalogue (OPAC): Most libraries have an On-Line Public Access Catalogue (OPAC) that lists all the books available in the library or the library system to which your library belongs. Some OPACs even list articles that would normally be found in the periodical index. (This is a growing trend.) Through OPAC you can gain access to all the books, videos, CD-ROMs, and computer software in your library's system that contain information relevant to your health care condition. To look for information on new titles that might not yet be in your library system, be sure to search Books in Print.

Interlibrary loan: Interlibrary loan is a system that allows you to borrow books not only from libraries outside of your state, but also from other countries around the world.

Vertical file collections: Many libraries have a file collection of pamphlets, government documents, and other materials that may not be listed in the OPAC.

Modem access: An increasing number of libraries offer direct access to their indexes through the Internet. This allows you to "call in" on your home computer, if you have a modem as part of your system, to gain entry into on-line services that can provide you with information.

Other important sources of information that are available in the library system in the U.S. include:

National Library of Medicine: The National Library of Medicine serves as the nation's primary medical information source. It provides on-line bibliographic searching capabilities that include Medline and the Index Medicus.

Medline Search (Medical Analysis and Retrieval Service On-line): Some public libraries and most university libraries offer access to "Medline Search," a service of the National Library of Medicine. Medline Search is a listing of nearly four thousand professionally published medical and health research journals. Given the vast amount of medical literature from around the world, it is not possible for Medline to include it all. In fact, many of the alternative medicine professional journals are not indexed in Medline although there is a growing trend to include more. Currently it is not considered a complete source of alternative medical treatments.

Index Medicus: Geared more to the professional and the scholar, Index Medicus is a printed index of three thousand of the journals included in Medline. It also includes definitions of medical terminology.

4. The Internet

Probably the most innovative and up-to-date way to learn your options is to use the Internet. Thousands of listings on the Internet specifically address the issues and techniques of alternative medicine through information sources, databases, and newsgroups.

The Internet is a worldwide network that connects millions of computers. Many of the computers on the Internet are capable of publishing or sharing information. The users of these systems can create documents that other users of the Internet can view by using their computers. In most cases it is possible for the viewer to print out the material on their computer screen.

There are several ways that information is published on the Internet:

The World Wide Web (WWW): The Web is the most popular for several reasons. Text, sounds, graphic images, and even movies can be integrated into a Web document, often referred to as a Web site or page. The documents are "hyper-textual," meaning that by pointing the computer's "mouse" at key words or phrases in the text of the document and "clicking," the Internet user will be able to access more detailed information on that word or phrase, often from other computers. This action is called "following a link."

HealthWorld Online is a website worth noting. It offers a vast amount of health information specifically about alternative medicine. Their information is reputed to be credible. In their first week of being online in March of 1996, sixty-seven thousand users took advantage of their services, and as a result Health-World Online was named one of the top forty websites in the world. Their Web address is: www.healthy.net.

UseNet News: UseNet News is a collection of newsgroups, each of which is a topically oriented stream of messages from users/readers all over the world with a shared interest in a theme or subject. Currently there are over two thousand newsgroups ranging on subjects as diverse as model airplanes to Bosnian culture. There is a large selection of newsgroups that focus on various alternative medical treatments. Some are listed by diagnostic conditions and others by the types of treatments.

Users/readers select the newsgroups they are interested in and read the postings from other participants. If they so desire, they can respond by "posting" something themselves, such as a question or a response to someone else's question or comment.

Public domain: On the Internet there are also "public domain" programs that are low cost or free, and legal to copy and distribute. These programs can be found for all types of information.

In order to use these resources, you need to have some form of access to Internet. Commercial networks such as America Online, Prodigy, or Compuserve provide access to Internet resources as well as have their own sources of information and discussion groups. Internet software is available at most computer stores, many book stores, and even some discount chains. This software has everything you need to set up your computer for the Internet. If you do not have an Internet-capable computer system at your disposal, your local library or community college may be your easiest access to the Internet.

See the Reference Section for additional specific Web addresses that may help you in learning your options for your particular health care needs.

5. Medical and health information service organizations

Because informed consumers want more detailed information than what most doctors have been willing, or able, to share with them, a new kind of "information broker" has emerged and is available to the public. These information brokers provide the public with various informational materials including research reports, books, pamphlets, as well as audio and video tapes covering a variety of health-related subjects and conditions.

Material on topics such as alternative options in health care treatment, the latest research data from around the world for particular health conditions, as well as networks of alternative practitioners and clinics are often provided. Some services educate their clients about new medical breakthroughs by either sponsoring conferences and symposia and/or publishing newsletters and news bulletins.

Interestingly, many of these information services were started by people who at one time faced their own health care crises and were frustrated by the lack of information they received about their conditions and treatment options. As a result of their personal trials, they created the information services they wished they'd had during their own crises.

One such highly respected organization is the World Research Foundation (WRF), in Sherman Oaks, California. Established by Steven and LaVerne Ross, the WRF is a worldwide, nonprofit health and environmental information network with regional offices in such diverse locations as India, China, Germany, as well as the United States.

Steven and LaVerne each faced a personal health care crisis. At the time, they were upset that they could not easily find the information they needed to make sound health care decisions. As a result of their experiences, they founded WRF on the belief that people have the right to be informed of all available treatments for diseases and should have the freedom to choose the treatment they want.

Services WRF offers to the public include free use of their extensive library facilities. For a nominal fee they will do an information search on your health condition. WRF says, "Library Searches contain information intended to introduce you to a range of alternative, complementary, and natural therapeutics for the specific illness or disease."[6] Their computer searches contain the latest research information from the National Library of Medicine's Medline database. Computer searches are available for over two hundred health conditions with the average report running 150 pages. In addition to their searches, they offer a quarterly newsletter, books and pamphlets, and have sponsored a number of informative and well-regarded conferences.

Another excellent information service is The Health Resource in Conway, Arkansas, founded by Janice Guthrie, whose story you read earlier in this chapter. The Health Resource's research reports contain information on both conventional and alternative therapies, as they believe it is important that patients be aware of all their treatment options. Each report is very well organized, easy to read, and addresses the client's diagnosis, age, sex, and any other possible critical factors. In addition to the searches, Health Resource offers an annual update on new treatments. As a free service to their clients, they also provide a newsletter and "news bulletins" of significant advances in particular treatments.

Terry Olsen, M.A., began Hermes Consumer Medical Search Service ("Hermes") after he lost his mother prematurely to cancer. He was disturbed by how few treatment options had been offered to him and his family and what little information was made available to them about techniques that might have eased her pain or treated her illness. Through exhaustive research, Terry discovered a myriad of resources for such information, from acupuncture for pain control, to radical, cutting-edge medical therapies being tried in the U.S. and abroad. Although it was too late for Terry to help his mother with the information sources he found, he knew that countless others could benefit from them. As a result, he founded Hermes.

Like the other information services described above, Hermes offers information searches that include conventional as well as alternative approaches to specific health care conditions. These searches consist of articles from journals, magazines, and newspapers; as well as protocols from the National Institutes of Health, personal stories, abstracts, adverse reactions to treatments, and information about medical devices.

"By sourcing and retrieving the most current medical information available," Olsen states, "we help you to become an active, informed co-participant in some of the most important decisions you may ever face: the choices you and your physician will make about your and your family's health care." [7] Becoming "an active, informed co-participant" is what each of the five steps in this book is designed to help you do.

When ordering a search from any information service, it is important to remember that you are receiving *information* that educates you about your health condition and options. *These services are not designed to give you medical advice.* For this reason, you must substantiate the accuracy of the information you receive. Always cross-check this information with other sources. Further in this chapter, you'll find criteria to help you verify that *any* information you gather is credible and valuable to you. In the

Reference Section of this book, you'll find a list of some of the best Health Information Service Organizations, what services they offer, at what price, and how to contact them.

6. Advocacy organizations and support groups

Often, people with particular medical diagnosis have joined together to emotionally support one another and to exercise their right to access medical information and treatments of their choice. Many of these groups support health care consumers during their healing and recovery process, particularly by educating them about unorthodox or unconventional approaches to treatment.

When learning your options, advocacy and support groups can be a valuable source of information. They can provide you with options you've never considered. During meetings you might hear from a member their first-hand experience of a controversial treatment.

Advocacy groups: As you learn your options for your particular health condition, be sure to search for advocacy groups representing your condition. Such groups exist on local, state, and national levels for many health conditions. Most are political in nature and try to influence legislation on the municipal, county, state, and federal levels by lobbying and demonstrating. They also offer educational programs for their members and the public. Many also offer legal advice on malpractice and malfeasance, as well as medical insurance investigation to assure that their members are getting all the benefits to which they are entitled. Advocacy groups in many cases also serve as a support group for their members. All have one thing in common: a commitment to insure that their members are getting all the helpful information available as well as the right to use the treatments of their choice.

One such organization is Patient Advocates for Advanced Cancer Treatment (PAACT, Inc.), which is considered one of the finest advocacy *and* support groups for victims of prostate cancer. In fact, it was PAACT that informed Michael about the treatment option that allowed his father to live another seven years, even though that treatment was not available or even legal in the U.S. at the time.

Lloyd J. Ney, the founder of PAACT, set up his organization in 1984 because he was extremely unhappy with his medical situation:

> I was diagnosed with prostate cancer. Because I didn't know a thing about it, I agreed to radiation — which was a disaster. From the radiation treatments my bladder distended four times its normal size, lost its elasticity, and now I sit here talking to you with a catheter and a bag on my abdomen. If that wasn't enough, after radiation therapy I had thirty-one bone tumors that I didn't have before radiation. When I found that out, I was disgusted and decided to find a therapy for the cancer that made sense to me. I found a great doctor in Canada. When I went to his office, I saw eighty people in the waiting room. I found out from the staff that 90 percent of those people were Americans! I decided right there to start something that would help all of us. I stood up and announced to all those people that I was starting a newsletter for people with prostate cancer and if they wanted to get this newsletter to give me their names. That was my first mailing list. [8]

Today PAACT has over twenty-seven thousand members and provides its members with information on *all* the treatment options for prostate cancer as well as a list of the doctors, clinics, and hospitals doing the latest, most effective, and least invasive treatments. PAACT also provides legal advice as well as insurance investigation as a member service.

Another advocacy organization is the AIDS Coalition to Unleash Power (ACTUP), which has gained much notoriety for its often dramatic demonstrations in support of AIDS awareness, education, and legislation. Some advocacy organizations such as ACTUP are quite controversial and provide access to treatments that are not approved by the FDA and are possibly illegal in the

U.S. Some are even conducting antidotal research studies with such treatments in the hopes of winning support for more formal studies. Advocacy groups are an excellent source of good health care information about your condition and options for treatment.

Support groups: Personal and professional therapeutic support, information services such as books, booklets, tapes and videos, as well as newsletters and conferences are just some of the services provided by illness support groups.

Many support groups are extremely empowering and valuable; unfortunately, others promote victimization. When considering a support group, be sure to evaluate what the support group is supporting. Joan Borysenko, Ph.D., says, "You don't need support in feeling like a victim, and if that's what you're getting, go elsewhere. A group, however, that supports the sharing of emotions and learning from illness is likely to have members who have researched both mainstream and alternative approaches." [9]

Many times support group members are well informed about the options of a particular disease and usually are more than happy to share their findings. In your effort to learn your options, find *healthy* support groups. They afford you an opportunity to gather relevant information as well as to receive personal and professional support from others with the same or similar diagnosis.

In the Reference Section of this book, you will find a list of some of the best advocacy organizations and support groups that are open to alternative medical treatments.

7. Professional organizations and trade associations

Most competent health care providers belong to at least one professional organization or trade association. The purpose of such groups is to further the cause of their members by setting standards for their profession or trade, provide advanced training and certification for the members, to further research into the health care treatments they represent, to protect their rights to use such treatments legally, as well as to educate the public about the efficacy of the health care treatments used by their members. Many of them publish journals with scientific research reports for various illnesses treated by the techniques advocated by the group.

The national association that represents acupuncturists, for example, is called the American Association of Oriental Medicine (AAOM). Founded in 1981, it is committed to supporting its members in maintaining high ethical standards for the practice of acupuncture and Chinese medicine. It is also committed to supporting legislation to regulate the licensing of acupuncture in all fifty states. Its members include individual acupuncturists, state and local professional acupuncture organizations, acupuncture schools and colleges, and research-related organizations. For its members, AAOM publishes a quarterly newsletter and sponsors an annual convention. For the public, it provides general information about acupuncture and a list of its members — all who have been screened for training, appropriate certification, and licensing.

The American Association of Naturopathic Physicians (AANP) nationally represents naturopathic physicians who have completed an in-depth four-year study of naturopathy at one of the three accredited naturopathic colleges. At this writing, naturopathic physicians are now licensed in twelve states to practice primary health care. AANP supports the efforts of its members to extend licensing privileges to additional states in the U.S. and also sponsors an annual convention for its members. For the public it offers a list of all its members and general information about naturopathic medicine for a small fee.

The American Holistic Health Association (AHHA) represents a variety of alternative providers who have similar practicing philosophies about health and well-being. AHHA's goal is to promote health and well-being through personal responsibility, considering the whole person (physical, emotional, mental, spiritual), wellness-oriented lifestyle choices, and active participation in personal health decisions and healing. AHHA offers to the public — at no charge — a variety of educational materials including: educational booklets; resource lists of professional referral organizations; information research services for specific diseases and chronic conditions; catalogs of self-help tools and educational opportunities; and an award-winning newsletter, A*h*H*a*!

As health care consumers, the educational and research efforts of these professional associations are of the most value to you. Many organizations have files full of research papers and information showing how well their treatments were in treating specific health conditions. Most will gladly share this information with you at no charge or for a nominal fee. A few will only share such data with their members. In that case, you need a professional health care provider who is a member of the organization to gain access to this information. (Remember, you have six other key sources for gathering information, so don't become too disappointed with closed files. It is probable that what they have "locked up" is readily available from one of the other six sources.)

In the Reference Section of this book, you will find a listing of many of the professional organizations and trade associations that advocate the use of alternative medical treatments.

The Three-Question Test for Complete and Dependable Health Care Information

When exploring each of these information sources, there are three questions to answer, which will help to ensure that you are getting *all* the information you need and that it is *accurate* and *credible*. They are:

1. What are the best treatments available in the world today for my health condition/diagnosis?

One of the downsides to the conventional medical system in the United States today is that many people believe it is the best medicine for every health condition that exists. While this is true for many health care conditions, it is certainly not the case for all. In addition to conventional medical treatments, there are many good alternative options in health care that are being used every day all over the world. They may be viable options in addition to those your M.D. has recommended. By thoroughly and success-fully participating in Step One and by utilizing the seven key sources to good health care information, you will be able to com-petently find all the answers for yourself.

2. Are those treatments proven effective?

This question is critical to answer if you are to make competent alternative health care choices. But sometimes it's a tricky call. For example, there are procedures and treatments based on good scientific research that are approved as effective by the World Health Organization and the European Economic Commu-nity (EEC) but are not accepted or approved by the Food and Drug Administration (FDA) in the United States.

In 1978 Germany set up a commission to study herbal treat-ments for illnesses. Over three hundred studies have been done, with two hundred and thirty showing positive results. Ginkgo Biloba ("Ginkgo") was one of the herbs studied. Based on the results of the study, it was approved by both the German govern-ment and the European Scientific Cooperative on Phytotherapy (ESCOP), which includes Belgium, France, Germany, Nether-lands, Switzerland, England, Greece, Ireland, and Italy. It was found to be an effective treatment for cerebrovascular insufficien-cy, memory loss associated with aging, early stages of Alzheimer's Disease, prevention and recovery from a stroke, tinnitus, poor cir-culation to the extremities, and intermittent claudication.

Still, the FDA has not approved the use of this herb for treat-ing these conditions. Because of this fact, your conventional doc-tor might say, "That is not a proven treatment," or "The FDA has not approved that as a treatment for your condition, so I would discourage you from using it." If this is the case, do not let your doctor's lack of knowledge stop your efforts to find the best treatment for yourself. Be a savvy health care consumer and take advantage of the vast amount of competent and reliable information from around the *whole* world. Do not just depend on information that only originates in the United States when determining what your health care options are for effective treatment.

3. How do I know if the information is reliable?

Regrettably, not all sources of health care information can be counted on to be accurate and unbiased. Well-meaning individuals as well as nefarious quacks abound in all walks of life. You as the health care consumer must practice "caveat lector: let the reader beware!" Unbridled enthusiasm over a particular remedy to your health problems can open the door to gullibility. On the other hand, being too critical can close your mind to viable options that could work for you.

Although there is no foolproof way to tell if the information is reliable, here are some important guidelines which can help:

- Seek sources of information that have been peer-reviewed and have stood the test of good scientific scrutiny.
- Consider using the Office of Alternative Medicine (OAM) Clearing House at the National Institutes of Health (NIH) to check the reliability of any information you have.
- Have your information reviewed and critiqued by an open-minded conventional doctor and/or other health care providers you trust and respect.
- Avoid treatments that are based on "secret formulas" or that claim miraculous cures or are based only on testimonials.
- Avoid products that are only advertised in the back pages of magazines, by direct mail, over the phone, in news-story-format newspaper ads, or infomercials and talk-show-format television ads.

WHAT'S NEXT

By using the strategies outlined in Step One, you now have access to all the information you need to make informed choices about your treatment options. Also, through the strategies listed in this chapter, you now know how to evaluate the information you find to be sure it is dependable and relevant to your health care situation. With this knowledge now yours, you've increased the chances that you will get the results you really want from your health care treatments.

As you begin Step Two: Get Good Referrals, you can move forward with confidence and know that you are really headed in the right direction for empowering yourself as a health care consumer. In Step Two, you will gather a list of good referrals who may be able to help you in your healing process. Your goal will be to find an alternative health care professional who can help you realize your goal of good health. As you do this, you will be one step closer to getting the best alternative health care.

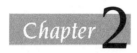

Chapter 2

STEP TWO: GET GOOD REFERRALS
Tapping the Networks

We spend more time shopping for a new car than for a health provider who may mean the difference between life and death for ourselves and our family.

— Bernie Siegel, M.D. [1]

An effective selection process is the key to locating a good health care professional. Getting high-quality referrals of good candidates is the best way to start that process. This chapter provides you with the information and know-how to get those high-quality referrals and to begin a selection strategy that can be used in hiring almost any alternative health care provider. Remember — they work for you!

When progressing through this second step, it is important to proceed with both eyes open. Alternative medical providers — just like M.D.'s — are trained to be informed health care consultants and highly skilled technicians. However, some are superb, others are average, and a few are downright dangerous.

Knowing how to choose a reliable alternative health care provider who is both responsible and well trained, rather than an unscrupulous and inadequately trained one, is critical. A poor choice can jeopardize your health and your life.

Although investing time to find a competent health care

provider is essential, it is rarely practiced. Time is precious, but so is your health and the health of your family. Invest your valuable time to make sure you get the best health care provider available. Using the strategies in the coming pages will help you get closer to health care provider(s) you'll want to work with.

An Anonymous Story: Deceivers Among Us

Several years ago, I was in a high-level position in city government and fighting multiple sclerosis. Conventional medicine did little to help my condition, so I tried alternative medicine. When I found some relief through a variety of alternative medical techniques, I enthusiastically shared my successes with my friends and family. I convinced many of them to try my alternative-care providers for their health care concerns. As a result, I think, at least one hundred people made appointments to see my alternative-care providers.

One of these providers was a colon therapist someone had recommended to me. Even before I had been to see her, I was encouraging my friends to see her. She was a very charismatic and charming woman. She had set up a colon therapy clinic in a very affluent part of town. The office was decorated to be a very pleasing and pleasant environment, which implied a competent and successful practice. Although this woman professed to care for her clients by supporting their healing, after seeing her for several appointments, I realized that money was her real priority.

After I stopped going to her, one of her employees later revealed several things to me. First, the employee told me that the owner personally trained all her employees and none of her staff had formal training in herbs, diet, or vitamin supplements. Also, she said that this woman routinely told her employees to recommend supplements and services that the clinic supplied — whether the client needed them or not.

I didn't know this woman was so unscrupulous when I recommended her to so many of my friends. I was horrified that someone like this woman could actually get away with such a deception. Fortunately, word "got around" about the unethical manner in which this woman was running her clinic, and the county closed her down. But not before I and many of my unsuspecting friends were collectively taken for thousands of dollars in supplements and services which were unnecessary and sometimes contraindicated.

I learned a hard lesson in this experience. I realized that my enthusiasm didn't serve me or my friends in this situation. Because of my naiveté, some of the people I care about were cheated out of their money and others were even physically harmed. I know now that checking to make sure a referral is trained and competent is really critical — for myself and for my friends.

WHAT YOU WILL LEARN IN THIS CHAPTER:
- *The seven key sources for getting good referrals*
- *Important questions to ask for getting good referrals*

The Seven Key Sources for Getting Good Referrals

When it comes to selecting a good alternative health care practitioner, it is best to start with a list of good referrals. To create that referral list, you may need to rely on more than one referral source. Relying just on family and friends may not give you the selection you need to find the right alternative-health professional.

Each of the seven key sources of referrals can potentially direct you to a good health care provider for your needs. By using more than one of them, you will increase your chances of finding the best alternative health care professional for your needs.

The seven key sources to getting good referrals are:

1. Family, friends, and colleagues
2. Local alternative practitioners
3. Local health-food stores

   4. Support groups

   5. Professional associations

   6. Alternative health care schools and colleges

   7. Referral services and advertisements

1. Family, friends, and colleagues

Right in your own home, neighborhood, or workplace, you'll find sources for good referrals. Seek out those family members, close friends, and colleagues you trust and respect, and who you know have had some experience with alternative medicine. Ask them to share with you the names of alternative health care professionals with whom they have had a positive and a successful health care experience. If you find a common name from several different sources, you may have found a good referral with potential. In truth, seeking the advice of friends and family is one of the most reliable ways to find a good clinician.

2. Local alternative practitioners

In each town or city, there exists an alternative practitioner network that is a natural outgrowth of the community. It is based on alternative health care providers' personal and professional reputation with one another. Generally, a good acupuncturist, if well-established in his or her practice, will know who the other good alternative practitioners are in town. These informal networks are a very valuable referral source. If you can just find one "good" alternative practitioner in your area, you may have found the key to many other good alternative health care providers. When you find such a person, ask him or her not only who he or she recommends, but also who *he or she* is treated by. By tapping into the alternative practitioner network, finding good referrals may be a fairly easy process.

3. Local health-food stores

Many health-food stores are a focal point for individuals involved in alternative medicine as part of their lifestyle. Not only do many of the practitioners frequent such stores, so do their patients/ clients. Because of this, most store employees are tapped into the local provider network and can lead you to good referrals.

Also, many health-food stores have a list of local alternative health care providers they recommend to their customers. Finally, be sure to look for a store bulletin board to see if any practitioners have put up cards or flyers about their services.

4. Support groups

Healing support groups are a great source for good referrals if the support group is geared toward getting healthier emotionally as well as physically. Many support groups provide a list of referrals they recommend. Also, in support meetings, you may hear a member share his or her personal experience about a health care provider that might spark your interest. Keep your eyes and ears open in a support group and you may get just the referral you've been hoping for.

5. Professional associations

As discussed in Step One, there are professional associations for many alternative treatment modalities. Most offer lists of alternative health care providers who are members of their association and practice in your area. More importantly, many of these associations screen for adequate training during membership evaluations. Although you won't get any details from the association about how a health care provider practices, you'll know that these referrals are adequately educated and licensed.

6. Alternative health care schools and colleges

Most alternative health care schools and colleges offer referral lists of their graduates. Like associations, you can be confident that the recommended health care providers have been adequately trained. Ask for graduates located in your area. Also, if the school or college is local to your area, request the names of alternative medical professors on staff who also practice locally.

7. Referral services and advertisements

Advertisements for all kinds of alternative health care providers are available in the yellow pages. The large ads do not, however, necessarily indicate a good health care professional. The more gimmicks the professional offers, the more caution is warranted when deciding to work with them. Dr. Alan Adams, vice president of Professional Affairs at Los Angeles Chiropractic College, states, "We did a study on the effectiveness in advertising for chiropractors. We found that advertising in the yellow pages with gimmicks and 'free services' does not build a practice for good chiropractors — word of mouth does." [2]

Referral services are advertised over the radio, on television, in magazines, and in the yellow pages. Generally, these systems list health care providers who pay to be recommended by the service. It is a way for health care professionals to add patients to their practice. Although these services do basic screening of licensure and education, a referral from these services does not insure a health professional of excellence. We recommend you screen these health care providers as closely as you screen your other referrals.

Important Questions to Ask for Getting Good Referrals

When getting a referral, you'll want to get as much information from your source as possible. Many times, with just a little extra information, you'll know immediately whether this referral has possibility for you or not.

Bernie Siegel, M.D., imparts valuable information when he encourages us to take time to "shop" for the right health care provider. It is critically important to explore details about a referral before assuming the provider is a good one.

Find out why specifically your contact recommends this health care provider. Keep in mind that their standard of care may or may not match yours. Also, the treatment that worked for him or her may not be appropriate for your own health care needs. Investigate and ask questions until you are personally satisfied that you have enough information to be complete. Probe for details!

Ask some or all of the following questions to the patient, health care professional, or organization offering you the referral. The answers will help you to know if this referral is worthy of follow-up.

Questions to ask a patient:

What was your purpose in seeking alternative medical treatment?

If their purpose is different than yours, this referral may not work for you.

What were your expectations?

Some people just want relief from uncomfortable symptoms. If you are looking to find the root cause of your physical problem and to really heal yourself, symptom relief may not be enough for you.

What is this health care provider's background?

Some patients have checked the educational training of their providers. If they can share that with you, you'll be one step ahead of the game.

What is their specialty or area of expertise?

Some providers are specially trained in treating specific health care problems. If this provider has a good track record in helping people with your health issue, this referral could have good potential.

Did this alternative medical professional listen attentively to you?

If good communication with your health care provider is important to you, a yes to this question can mean a good referral.

Did he or she effectively explain your condition and recommended treatment?

Getting all the relevant detail from a health care provider can indicate a high quality professional.

Can you get to this health care provider quickly by appointment or by phone?

A provider who responds quickly to his or her patients can indicate a conscientious professional who respects his or her clients.

What specific results did you get from the treatment? After how many treatments?

This is a very important question. If this person received good results in a reasonable amount of time, it is a great indicator of a good referral. If, however, this person received minimal results after an extraordinary amount of time and money, this should indicate that perhaps this practitioner is not right for you.

Did you feel the professional charged you fairly for his or her time, and for recommended supplements?

A good health care provider is not measured by his or her fees. Some excellent health care providers are reasonable in fee and high in competence. If, however, your contact feels he or she was charged unethically, you need to take this information into consideration.

Questions to ask a health care professional:

How do you know this provider?

If the health care professional knows the provider professionally this person may have a good indication of the provider's skills and competence. If, however, the professional's affiliation with the provider is more personal, you might not get an accurate reading of what this provider can offer you.

Have you had personal experience(s) with this provider that indicates to you that he or she is good at his or her profession?

If this provider actually works on the professional, you'll get a very clear picture of how this provider works and his or her strengths and weaknesses.

What is this health care provider's specialty or area of expertise?

Again, *specific* expertise can indicate this provider has the skills to help you with your *specific* health care problem.

Would you go to this provider for your health care needs? If so, why?

If this professional wouldn't go to this provider, you'll want to know why.

What kind of reputation does this provider have with his or her peers?

You'll want to know how this provider rates among his or her co-workers, so monitor the response to this question closely.

Do you know his or her training?

Some will. If so, it will save you the time and effort of checking the candidate's education.

Tell me about this person's personality.

An advanced look at what kind of personality characteristics this provider has might indicate if this provider is right for you.

Is he or she easy to talk to?

Again, the answer to this question shows you whether this personality is a match for you.

Is this the kind of provider who could feel comfortable in partnership with a patient?

If you're interested in having a partnership with your provider, this answer may tell you if this is possible.

Questions to ask an association or educational facility:

Can you verify that this person has completed the necessary education and has a degree and/or is certified?

They should be able to give you the years of study completed as well as date of graduation.

Has this provider been reprimanded by his or her board or any certifying or educational body for any reason?

This is important information to get. If they have been reprimanded, get the details. A well-founded reprimand can mean that you should cross this referral off your list.

It is important to remember that you are the one who determines which questions are important to have answered. The key is to make sure that all of the questions that are important to *you* are answered to your satisfaction.

WHAT'S NEXT

Step One gives you the important information you need in order to know what *all* the treatment options are for your health care condition. Possibly you learned about treatments that you've never even heard of. Not only that, you probably learned information about your health care condition you did not know before.

In Step Two, by using the "seven key sources to getting good referrals," you gathered enough names to create a list of practitioners who probably offer some of the treatment options you are considering.

Now that you have completed Step Two, you have a list of referrals with good potential. You can feel confident that you've tipped the scales in your favor and that you are now just a few steps away from finding a health care provider who you'll want to work with. In the next chapter, Step Three: Screen the Candidates, you will use the information you gathered in the previous steps to determine if the health care providers on your referral list have the appropriate training you need, the "bedside manner" you prefer, as well as any other criteria that are important to you. By actively participating in Step Three, you will be able to select with confidence those alternative health care providers you would like to interview. By working through these steps you'll move closer to receiving the kind of alternative medical treatment you want. 🔥

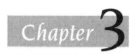

STEP THREE: SCREEN THE CANDIDATES

If Only All Health Care Providers Were Created Equal

Walking through a doctor's door without taking charge of the selection process is playing Russian roulette with your health.

– Lawrence Horowitz, M.D. [1]

In this chapter, the alternative health care provider's office staff will become an invaluable information source to you. Without spending a penny in fees, you can get a more in-depth picture about this provider's personality, his or her expertise, his or her educational training, and which associations or professional organizations he or she belongs to. From this information, as well as the additional information you will garner from asking some very specific, well-targeted questions, you will gain greater certainty as to whether this candidate could be your health care provider.

You might wonder why you wouldn't just approach the health care practitioner first. It is important to use the staff as an information source to *screen* the candidates, because you do not want to pay a provider to answer questions the staff could have answered for free. Even worse, if you don't screen the candidate, you may find yourself paying the provider an interview fee just to discover that he or she is not the right health care practitioner for you. Not only is this a waste of your money, it's a waste of your time and energy.

So, as a preliminary step to finding the right health care partner, be prepared to ask questions pertinent to your needs. In the following pages, you'll find many good questions to choose from.

Amanda's Story: If Only I'd First Asked Some Questions!

A few years ago, I was thrown by a horse, and the way I landed damaged my jaw. Within a week, my jaw was going out of socket two to three times during a meal. I needed some help. I contacted a trusted friend who happened to also be an excellent chiropractor. He had been very effective in treating other complications from the accident, and suggested that I make an appointment immediately to see a particular dentist whom he highly recommended. This dentist, an authority on jaw problems, was an "expert witness" in court cases involving jaw injuries. Feeling confident that he could help me, I made an appointment the next day. This dentist rearranged his schedule so I could be tested and treated immediately.

When I arrived, I was whisked into a treatment room. The dentist entered, introduced himself, and said that after the testing we would meet again to discuss treatment options. His assistant hooked me up to a machine that measured the volume level of the "click" when my jaw went out of joint — the louder the click, the worse the condition. As she measured the first of a series of "clicks," she asked the dentist to come into the room. He asked me to move my jaw so that the "click" happened again. He was amazed when he heard the noise. Calling several other assistants into the room, he said, "You folks ought to hear this one. I've never seen a condition this bad before!" In paraded another three assistants to hear the dentist elaborate about my condition. He referred to me as the "patient" or "this case" — never by my name. Suddenly, in this personal testing session, I became the show in the center ring.

Next, I was hooked up to a machine which electrically forced my jaw to snap open and shut — to stretch my traumatized jaw muscles back to normal elasticity. I was appalled as the assistant turned on the machine. Besides the humiliating feeling of having my jaw involuntarily snapped open and shut, I could feel my muscles being further traumatized by the treatment. I knew this was not for me.

As soon as the assistant unhooked me, I left, knowing that I would never return again. I realized that I should have gathered more information before the visit, but at the time, screening a medical professional before agreeing to treatment never occurred to me.

After a week of serious research into effective non-invasive treatments for my jaw, and screening several candidates, I found a compassionate, superbly trained orthodontist. I shared with him my experience with the dentist and explained the treatment and testing that had occurred. The orthodontist commented that the treatment I described was very outdated and was not effective for long-term success. He recommended a less invasive, more effective treatment plan which I tried with great success. This orthodontist was respectful, considerate of my feelings, answered all my questions — and best of all, gave me the results I wanted.

Now I know how important it is to take the time to ask the right questions when shopping for a good health care provider. I can't emphasize enough how critical it is to screen the professional and his or her treatments before you agree to let him or her practice on you.

WHAT YOU WILL LEARN IN THIS CHAPTER:
- *How to get valuable information without scheduling an appointment*
- *Questions to ask the health care provider's staff when screening the candidates*

How to Get Valuable Information Without Scheduling an Appointment

At this point, you can take the list of good referrals that you gathered in Step Two and investigate them further by arranging to speak with the appropriate staff person at his or her office. Find out who the best staff person is to answer your questions and the best time for you to speak with that person.

Keep in mind that running a health care clinic can be challenging work — the office staff is not only juggling patients and phone calls but the employer too! When placing your call, tell the receptionist that you're considering making an appointment with the provider; however, you have several questions you would like answered first. Whom should you talk to?

When you get to that person, ask him or her if this is a good time to ask your questions, or if he or she would prefer to schedule a phone appointment at a more convenient time. Posing this question lets the staff person know that you respect his or her time and helps to ensure that you'll get the staff member's full attention so that he or she can give you satisfactory answers to your questions.

Remember that there may be certain questions that the staff prefer the practitioner answer him- or herself. This is not an uncommon practice, especially when addressing the technical, personal, and detail-oriented issues of a particular treatment or specific health care need.

Also consider that a clinic has a personality just as a provider does — and how the office staff answers your questions can provide great insight into how you will be treated as a patient. If the staff is open and helpful, the provider is also probably open and helpful. "A healthy clinic is one where you can get straight, honest answers," Dr. Christiane Northrup, author and founder of the Women to Women clinic, elaborates. "You don't want to feel that the staff's job is to protect the health care professional. If you have a sense that the staff is being an armor for the doctor, that isn't good. I feel that the staff should be an extension of the doctor. They should be helping all the way along the line."[2]

Some provider's offices are healthy and support your healing; others are unhealthy and can compromise your healing. John E. Upledger, Doctor of Osteopathy, and founder and president of The Upledger Institute says:

> If I ever hear of a staff member being curt or uncompassionate with a patient, they are most likely going to get fired. It is imperative that we have an excellent staff because they can make such a difference for the patients. For instance, a woman who works here at the office developed breast cancer a year ago. She first went to an oncologist whose nurse was just brutal. This woman would say, "Oh, the chemotherapy is making me sick." The nurse would retort, "Well, what do you expect?" — then tell her that her insurance was behind in payments and that she better do something about it. Not surprisingly, the woman did poorly with this doctor. Then she found another physician who treated her with compassion — and so did his staff. Six months ago I wouldn't have given two cents for her ability to survive. Now she looks like she's got it made. Same medical treatment as the first doctor; it was the emotional treatment that made the difference.[3]

Bernie Siegel, M.D., also emphasizes the importance of the staff. "I think the staff plays an incredibly important role," he says. "In most cases, the nurses and the staff do all the talking and loving and hugging. I hear that from lots of nurses. I know a person who swears she was saved by my secretary. This woman called up my secretary, who happened to also have had cancer three times. The woman said, 'I'm supposed to die.' The secretary said, 'What do you mean?' The woman said, 'The lady just gave me the statistics. I'm supposed to die.' My secretary said, 'Look, statistics are for dead people. You're not dead.' The woman wrote to me and said, 'Your secretary saved my life by telling me that. It changed everything for me!'"[4]

If you are ill, support from your health care provider and his or her staff can make the difference between a good recovery and a poor recovery. Respect yourself by insisting on respect from your provider and his or her staff.

Questions to Ask the Health Care Provider's Staff When Screening the Candidates

The following is a list of questions you may want to have answered when you screen your potential health professional. You may not feel that they all relate to you, so choose the ones that will give you the information you feel you need. The answers to these questions will help you feel informed when choosing your alternative health care provider.

If the support staff is unavailable to answer all of these questions, you can certainly apply some of these questions to the actual practitioner interview, which is explored in Step Four.

What are the alternative health care provider's areas of expertise?

Most health care professionals have an affinity for working with a certain set of health care problems, specific alternative medical technique(s), or a certain part of the population (i.e., men, women, children, older adults). Asking the professional's areas of expertise can help indicate if this health care provider can be a match for you.

What success has this alternative doctor had in treating patients with physical problems similar to mine?

If you have a specific condition to correct, knowing the health care professional's track record with your particular condition will be a significant factor in deciding whether to work with him or her. Ask to have satisfied patients call you and relate their success stories working with this doctor. Generally, if patients are happy with their results, they are apt to share them.

What techniques or treatments will the provider use to treat my health condition?

Many times the staff knows the treatments used to help specific health problems. If they do, you can research the effectiveness of the types of treatment before you even meet the health care candidate.

Can you provide me with literature about the health care provider's educational background and philosophy of treatment?

Marketing the skills of the health professional is one of the requirements of running a successful clinic. Therefore, it is likely the office provides a description of this health care professional's philosophy of treatment, a brief history of his or her educational background, the techniques he or she uses, and sometimes articles he or she has authored. Asking for a copy of all the health professional's literature, including a copy of his or her license or diploma, will assist you in determining if this provider of alternative medicine is in support of your own beliefs about medicine and patient care. If, by chance, the health professional does not offer information in printed form, ask someone on the staff to tell you over the phone about the professional's philosophy of treatment, education, treatments methods, and any articles he or she has authored.

How long has the doctor/health care provider been in practice?

Although health professionals are well trained in school, the ones who have vast clinical experience may be more effective in treating the condition you would like to improve. There are exceptions, however, to this line of thinking. Sometimes health professionals who have been treating the same way for many years may have grown rigid in their ability to learn the latest techniques for your condition. Be sure that this alternative health care provider's method of treating your condition is the most up-to-date, the most effective, and the least drastic to you. You can cross-check this information by using one or more of the seven key sources to good health care information in Step One.

Will the provider allow a family member or friends to be with me in the treatment room?

If you need a friend with you for moral support, or someone to be there to understand what you will need later for care at home, let this provider know. Alternative health care providers, just like conventional health care providers, should have nothing to hide.

Can you describe the doctor's "approach" with his or her patients? In other words, can you describe his or her bedside manner?

Listen for how much time the doctor spends with his patients. Does the doctor answer patient's questions in a manner that a patient can understand? Is the style cold and stiff or open, warm, and friendly? Does the doctor communicate clearly? The answers may indicate to you if you will feel comfortable and supported by this alternative health care physician.

What associations does the health care provider belong to?

Associations not only indicate that this health care provider is accepted by his or her professional peers, it also can indicate this individual's philosophy of medicine, as well as his or her willingness to keep abreast of continuing changes within the profession. Let's say you are interested in working with a holistic M.D. who acknowledges the mind/body connection. Knowing that the doctor is a member of the Society of Behavioral Medicine indicates he or she not only appreciates the mind/body connection in healing but probably is also knowledgeable about many of the latest findings and techniques. Remember to ask for the phone numbers of the associations.

How are emergency calls or appointments handled?

If you have an emergency during the night or on weekends, you'll want the expertise of the health care provider who is overseeing your care. Make sure you can get to your provider when you might need him or her most.

Can I see him or her during evenings or weekend hours?

For many people with work or family commitments, free time is evenings and weekends. If this provider cannot see you during this time, you may need to make special arrangements so you can see him or her.

Where is the provider located?

Knowing you'll be spending a lot of time traveling to a provider may help you decide not to hire this one.

Is the provider available for consultation by phone?

Many times a patient has questions that require an answer, yet do not necessitate an office visit. Make sure this provider will take the time to answer your questions in a reasonable amount of time by return phone call.

Does the provider usually get behind on his schedule? If so, how long would I usually have to wait for my appointment?

Some health care professionals are almost always behind on their schedules. This can be frustrating if you aren't prepared in advance. If you know, however, that this provider will be a half-hour late or more, you can be prepared for this wait by bringing a book or other activity.

Does this health care provider set up consultations with prospective patients?

Most will. Ask how much the fee will be. If this is your first experience with this health care provider, ask for a fifteen-minute meeting. The fee will be much lower. Generally, you will know quickly whether you like this professional, whether you can work with him or her, and if you have confidence in this person's skills. If the meeting is successful, you can set a longer consultation at a later date. If you don't like this health care provider, you won't be obligated to an uncomfortably long session, nor will you be billed for one.

Generally how long is a first appointment?

If your first appointment with a health care provider is fifteen minutes, then you'll know this professional won't be doing a very detailed medical history or be able to take the time you may need to get answers to your questions or to explain treatment options. A usual first appointment is about an hour. If this is not the case, look elsewhere.

What is the fee structure, your policy with insurance, and how much can I expect to pay on my first visit, including tests, supplements, and prescriptions?

First visits can be astronomical in price. It is better to know what to expect than to be surprised. The staff may not be able to give an exact price until the health care provider actually sees you, but they should be able to give you a range based on the professional's "new patient" procedures.

They should also be able to share with you a breakdown of that initial fee. Find out exactly how much the doctor charges per hour and any additional fees which the provider will expect you to pay and what they are for. It also is a good idea to know before you make an appointment whether the provider will bill your insurance company or whether you are expected to pay the fee out-of-pocket, submit your own forms, and wait for your own reimbursement. Also, find out if they know if your insurance carrier will cover the treatments you will be receiving. If the staff has billed your carrier previously, they'll know whether or not reimbursement is likely.

Will the staff help me with my medical insurance forms and submit them?

These days insurance forms can be confusing and tedious. The staff of an alternative medical clinic will usually know better than the patients the strategy for getting reimbursement for insurance. Make sure you can use their expertise and their help.

Will the provider allow installment payments?

Because many alternative treatments are not yet covered by insurance carriers, most fees are out-of-pocket and can quickly add up to a hefty amount. Many alternative providers are aware of this difficulty and are willing to make payment plans so that you can get the care you need and they can receive their fees in a timely manner.

Is the provider willing to discuss fees?

If you need care, but are short on funds, don't be shy about asking to negotiate fees. Many alternative providers will work with you. But you have to ask!

Is your office near public transportation or public parking?

If you are disabled or hurt, make sure you won't have to walk blocks to reach this provider's office. If you need some assistance to get to the office, let the staff know. They may be able to assist you.

Finally, if you find you are not sure about a particular candidate after speaking to the office staff, here are a few questions to ask yourself that can help you clarify what, if any, next steps are appropriate for these uncertain candidates:

Does this health care professional seem to have the skills and the experience to give you the results you're seeking?

If they do not, you won't feel confident in his or her ability to help you and you should cross this candidate off your list. If the person is competant but you're hesitating because of character flaws, you need to decide if his or her competency is more important than your personality compatibility.

Do you think he or she has a personality you can work with?

Sometimes a personality cannot be fully described by a third party. You may need to meet face to face with a provider to know if you can work together. Think about setting up just a ten-minute meeting with a provider. Your gut instincts can tell you instantaneously if this provider is for you.

Are you interested in meeting the person to see if he or she is right for you?

Possibly you feel curious about someone. You might wonder what he or she is like. If you have the time and money, humor your curiosity and meet with this provider. You may be pleasantly surprised to find just the provider you'd hoped you'd find.

WHAT'S NEXT

Congratulations! By screening your candidates, you've just narrowed your list of candidates to a select few whom you'd like to meet. You're only one step away from the alternative health care practitioner with whom you will want to develop a health care partnership.

The time and the energy you've used to gather information about your health care options and the candidates is about to pay off. With all this credible information, you're about to come face to face with the provider(s) who just might help you realize your health care goals. Over the course of Step Four, you'll be asking these candidates questions that indicate if you can build a working, active partnership with this provider. Know that you are just one step away from creating the partnership that will help you reach your health goals. You have come a long way and are to be commended for your persistence and commitment. What you have done for yourself so far is no less than inspiring!

Chapter 4

STEP FOUR: INTERVIEW THE PROVIDER

Making the Most of the Facts and Your Instincts

The doctor-patient relationship is one of the most delicate and intricate human-to-human relationships that exists. It contains much magic, mystery, and wonder. This complexity is why the intuition and feeling that the patient has for a doctor is so vastly important. The choice of physician can never be decided by an algorithm, a decision-making flow chart, or on the basis of answers to some 'ten key questions.' We should use our rational facilities in sizing up a prospective doctor and ask the questions; but we have hearts as well as heads — which in this circumstance may be more important.

— Larry Dossey, M.D. [1]

Participating in Step Four gives you a personal experience with the health care professionals on your list of screened candidates. To successfully interview these health care providers, you must ask the right questions and use your own gut instincts to get a feel of who these people are and if they are right for you. These interviews will provide you with valuable data to help you determine which of these professionals you will want to work with.

You may wonder why getting in front of the professional is important at this point. You have checked their credentials and treatments. What if you're excited about this provider and just want to make an appointment? Be patient just a little while longer. Private time with this provider can save you time and effort in the long run.

Michael had an experience several years ago when a family member raved about an orthopedic M.D. The relative told him how highly respected and successful this doctor was. It sounded reasonable that this doctor could help with a shoulder injury Michael had just received. He was looking forward to seeing the doctor, so he made an appointment instead of requesting an interview. When this doctor met him in what seemed like a cubbyhole with little privacy, the doctor was rude, condescending, and completely disregarded Michael's perspective on his injury. Michael left the office no closer to a solution to his shoulder problem than when he arrived and $100 poorer.

This next step requires that you make the effort to visit your candidate and perhaps pay a small fee for his or her time. In the long run, it's a good investment.

Robert's Story: Only the Best for My Mother

Several years ago, my mother was diagnosed with a brain tumor that was going to have to be surgically removed. Because I knew my mother would be in significant danger during the surgery, I wanted to do everything I could to insure that my mother survived. I knew nothing about brain surgery at the time, but decided I should get informed about the procedure the doctors would perform on my mom. That way I could interview surgeons with some degree of competence. I realized that in order to do that I needed to know as much as the surgeons knew about the operation. So I went to the library at Stanford University and studied the procedure until I felt that I understood the whole technique.

While I was doing the research, I found some valuable information available to anyone. Hospitals are rated annually for specific surgical procedures — how many successes and how many failures [deaths]. That information was a real key. I knew if I found the hospital with the highest success rate for this type of brain surgery, I could maximize the successful results of my mother's surgery.

Also, because of my work as a scientist, I was around the medical field enough to know that there are good doctors and bad doctors; there are good surgeons and bad surgeons. I was determined to find the best one to do the job. I interviewed about fifteen surgeons and every time I talked to one, I learned more about the surgical procedure. That helped me to refine my interviewing method.

In my interviews, I found that several of the surgeons would have made mistakes — used the wrong anesthetic or technique. I am convinced that my mom wouldn't have survived those surgeries. Then I found a surgeon who I knew was the right one. He had significant experience in performing this surgery. His record of successful surgeries was impressive. From his answers to my questions, I knew he would be using the correct anesthetic, the best technique. Obviously he was very bright. I just knew he was the man for the job.

I can say that I was pretty nervous during her surgery but, just as I hoped, she came through with flying colors. No mistakes were made during the procedure and she recovered fairly quickly.

I'm really glad I took the time to find the right surgeon for my mother. I am convinced that she is alive today because of the information I gathered during my research and because I took control of the situation by interviewing each and every surgeon until I found the right one for my mom.

WHAT YOU WILL LEARN IN THIS CHAPTER:
- *Preparing for the interview: A question to ask yourself first*
- *Strategies for making the most of your interview time*
- *Questions you need answered to make a competent decision about treatments with the provider*
- *Making a choice: Is this the one for you?*

Preparing for the Interview: A Question to Ask Yourself First

Now that you have learned your options, received good referrals, and screened the candidates, you have at your disposal a body of reliable information about your health care condition, viable treatment options, and verified information about several alternative health care providers that might work for you.

Now you are about to interview the practitioners. In order to make the most of the interview, you need to answer the following question first:

What kind of personality do you need in a health care professional?

Superbly trained health care providers come in a wide range of personalities. Some have nurturing bedside manners and are compassionate and sensitive with their patient/clients. Some are cold rationalists who don't really care about the thoughts and feelings of their clients. Others are somewhere in the middle. Being human, all medical professionals are subject to changes in temperament at times depending on the situation, their mood that day, your personality, and the chemistry, or lack thereof, between the two of you.

A health care professional's personality does not necessarily indicate that provider is competent. You can find excellent care from each character extreme as well as from health care provider's in between.

Take a personal inventory now. Which personality fits best with your needs?

Leonard Wisneski, M.D., medical director for the Marriott Corporation, believes the quality of emotional support from a health care provider is important. "I personally feel that the humanistic qualities of a health care provider are equally important as the expertise of the physician," he says. "I feel it is imperative that a patient feel very comfortable with his or her physician as a human being. One must feel comfortable that enough time is being allotted, that all questions are being answered, and that all fears are being allayed. That is a tall order. But due to the number of available health care providers today, I feel that the consumer really should demand that and should expect that."[2]

When Dr. Larry Dossey, author and executive editor of *Alternative Therapies*, was a patient, he had a different set of emotional needs than Dr. Wisneski described. "I feel that I have a very strong spiritual resourcefulness," he says. "I'm a very self-reliant person when it comes to dealing with the higher aspects of being alive. So when I had a ruptured disk in my back and had to choose a surgeon, I didn't want spiritual or emotional support from my doctor. In some sense, I would have seen that as a kind of intrusion. So I chose a very rational, very cold, intellectual, highly skillful, superbly trained neurosurgeon. I picked him because I felt I could take care of my inner needs and handle all of that. I wanted him to come at my problem from rational competence. So I saw it as a complementary thing."

Dr. Dossey is correct when he concludes, "We all don't need the same doctor. Thank God there are different types of doctors. It gives us a chance to match up according to what feels right for us."[3]

However, most people's ideal health care provider is closer to what Dr. Wisneski describes: sort of TV's Dr. Marcus Welby — a professional who is compassionate, intelligent, highly skilled, inspirational, listens attentively to the patient, is consummately knowledgeable about all the details of the physical problem, and gives the client just what he or she needs to get him or her back to perfect health.

Obviously, such a doctor would be what most of us would like. But Dr. Marcus Welby, or a provider just like him, may not be available. So, what if you are faced with a health care professional who can be *almost* everything you need? If that is the case, it is important that you be clear about your needs — all your needs. You may have to give up some of your ideals of the perfect health care provider for you.

Consider this: You are in a health crisis where the health care professional you need most is a superbly skilled, highly egotistical surgeon with a bad temper. Even if emotional support was very important to you, a less skilled, yet compassionate surgeon may not do the job you really need. If that was true, you would be wise to reconcile yourself to the health care provider your body needs and find other resources for emotional/spiritual support.

Determine which *personality* traits of your health care provider are negotiable and which are not. Knowing this will assist you in making optimal use of your interview.

Strategies for Making the Most of Your Interview Time

The interview is the time to ask in-depth questions of the health care professional. It is your time to discover if you can confidently work with this person. Dr. Larry Dossey says, "I think in the first visit, one can gain an intuitive feel as to whether this is really going to work or not. If it doesn't feel right after the first visit, then one ought to move on. It is your money." [4] Be sure to make the most of every minute to evaluate this professional. In most cases, you are paying for that privilege.

Here are some strategies to help make your interview a success:

Use your intuition when sizing up this professional.

Your own intuition, or "gut instinct," is a very valuable tool in determining which provider is right for you. All of us have within us a deep resource of wisdom that goes beyond the rational mind. It is wise to use *all* your brain — the rational and the intuitive — when choosing a health care provider.

You may get immediate insight in the first thirty seconds of your meeting; first impressions are many times accurate intuitive insights into people and situations. Possibly you may just "know" by the end of your meeting if this provider is right for you or not. You might just have a nagging anxious feeling that is trying to tell you, "No!" You would be wise to trust that feeling. Also, watch for messages that may come in other ways, such as dreams and fantasies, or possibly from coincidence and serendipity. Whatever your intuitive insights, make sure you take them into consideration when deciding on this or other health care providers.

Keep the details straight.

To help you to remember all the questions you'd like to have answered by the health care provider, bring a list of those questions with you to the interview. This will help to keep you focused on what is important to you. Having a set number of questions also lets your provider know you won't be taking more time than you requested.

Another point: If you think you'll have trouble remembering the details of the meeting, consider bringing along a tape recorder or a friend. Either one can help you relive the details of your meeting with clarity. Dr. Christiane Northrup, author of *Women's Bodies, Women's Wisdom* (Bantam, 1994), explains, "Sometimes an interview can mean high stress for a prospective patient/client. I love it when they bring a friend. It diffuses some of the tension, but also the friend can remind the prospective client of details of the meeting which were important but were forgotten. If the provider is upset that you have brought a friend, you can be sure that you've got the wrong provider. I also often suggest my clients bring in a tape recorder if they feel they need to go over all the data later."[5] If you do not want to bring a tape recorder, then take detailed notes.

Be courteous, comfortable, and frank during your meeting.

A first meeting with a health care professional can induce some anxiousness. In spite of this, attempt to rise above the tension. If you act either defensively or aggressively during this interview, the provider is likely to be less open and less friendly than you'd like. Help the provider feel relaxed and comfortable by being the same yourself. It's amazing how much you can influence the tone and the content of this meeting by acting in a manner that brings the best out of the provider you are meeting with.

In addition, you'll want to share your information and ask your questions with confidence. This will cue the provider that you respect your thoughts and feelings and he or she should too.

Be sure to describe clearly what you know about your condition.

Let the provider know that you consider yourself an educated person and that you have attempted to understand your condition through a medical diagnosis as well as research. Share with him or her what you have learned and why you trust this information. The provider will try to gage if the information that *you* offer is worth exploring.

Share your information with competence and confidence — if you are confident about it. If you are sharing information you aren't yet sure about, make sure the professional knows that too. A provider is more likely to take *your* information and recommendations seriously if he or she knows you are familiar with your condition and are able to discuss it intelligently.

Share with the professional that you have educated yourself about some of the treatment options.

Let this professional know that you have also done some homework about the available treatment options. Make sure that you add that you are interested in learning more — especially what treatment options he or she recommends.

At this point, be sure to gage their reaction to your "being informed." Does your being informed seem to threaten him or her? If you think this might be true, but you aren't sure, ask him or her point blank, "Are you uncomfortable with the fact that I am actively learning about my treatment options?" The provider should let you know very quickly if this is an issue. If it is, this is clearly a negative mark for this provider.

Let the health care provider know which techniques you would like to try and why.

Acknowledging that you are not an expert in medical matters, tell this provider which techniques have gotten your attention and why you think they might work for you. Again, you need to be clear about which treatments you have some degree of certainty about and which ones you are open to learning more about. If the provider seems to brush off treatment options that you *know* through your research have a good chance of helping you, that is also a negative mark for a provider — especially if they are not willing to see for themselves the research data you have found.

Respond to the provider's recommendations honestly.

The greatest favor you can do for both yourself and your health care provider during a consultation is to be honest. The best relationships, professional and personal, are built on honesty. If you don't agree with what the provider is telling you or, more importantly, what he or she recommending you *do*, you must respectfully tell this person how you feel. Dr. Dossey suggests, "This is certainly not a situation for hidden agendas. To play a 'yes' game with an alternative medical doctor when you believe the total opposite of what the doctor believes, poisons the power of the relationship right off." [6]

Agreeing to therapies and medical philosophies you do not have confidence in will also undermine the potential of the provider/patient relationship. Not only that, agreeing to treatment you do not believe in can adversely affect your chances of successful treatment.

Pace the interview and remember to listen.

Remember to watch the clock and to pace yourself. If you make an appointment for fifteen minutes, limit the visit to that. Also, make sure you do not spend all your time telling the health care professional about your condition. Dr. Dossey says, "Most patients who come to interview me forget about time. Many get wound up in the details of their illness and go on and on. If you spend all the time talking, what can you learn about the health care provider? 'Interview' by definition is two-way — talking and listening on the part of both parties." [7]

Fifteen minutes isn't very long. So keep in mind that the interview is just that: a time to get a feel, to get the sense of rightness or wrongness about coming back and going further with this provider.

Questions You Need Answered to Make a Competent Decision About Treatments with the Provider

By the time you leave the interview, your goal is to have a clear sense about how you feel about this provider's treatment options for your condition. And, whether or not you feel comfortable working with them specifically. A provider doesn't have to know all the solutions to your health care problem, but if you have a strong sense that he or she would take you down a "wrong road" — away from the health care goals you have in mind — you'll want to know that as soon as possible.

Here are some good questions to ask to help you determine if this is the right provider and treatment for you:

Which tests, treatments, and techniques have worked for other patients with my diagnosis?

This is where your research can be very valuable. If the provider gives you treatments that you *know* have little or no effectiveness for your condition, you'll question the competence of this professional. On the other hand, if he or she mentions treatment options that looked promising in your research, you'll feel more confident that this provider could help you get good results.

Can you provide me with evidence that the treatment you are recommending is the least drastic and most effective treatment available for my condition?

The best evidence a health care professional can provide you is competent research findings. Many alternative treatments, however, have not yet been thoroughly researched. In that case, anecdotal evidence of successful results is the next best thing.

How long will it be before I can expect results?

Many times people continue treatments far too long — despite the fact that they aren't seeing any positive responses from them. Find out in this initial meeting in what amount of time can you reasonably expect to see a positive improvement in your condition.

How will we know the treatment is working?

Some treatments make the condition worse first before they make it better. For example, homeopathic treatments sometimes involve a period in which the very symptoms you are seeking relief from become more aggravated for a certain period of time before permanent relief is achieved. Make sure you know how the symptoms will progress as you move toward your goal of better health. Also, you will want to know how the provider will monitor your progress, and particularly what indicators he or she will be looking for.

Are there any side effects?

This is a very important question. Side effects can greatly affect your quality of life by for example, creating drowsiness or even pain. They can even cause iatrogenic diseases (diseases created by medical treatments). Find out if and how this treatment will affect your health: in what way and to what degree.

Will there be any follow-up treatments?

Many times a provider will do treatment programs which entail several treatments together or in succession. Make sure you know how many treatments the provider is recommending, in what time frame they will be administered, and how they all work together.

How much will my treatment program cost?

You'll need to know how much the supplements/drugs will cost as well as how many office visits you'll need and at what cost. Also, find out if you need to buy any special devices or special foods. As we've stated, there can be a vast range of fees from one provider to another — even among providers who practice in the same system of medicine. For example, a chiropractor we work with charges $35 per visit and usually prescribes about $30 in supplements per visit. He will also see a child under three years of age at no charge. Another chiropractor we know charges $150 per hour and usually prescribes between $100 and $200 in supplements per visit. We have also heard of two different chiropractors in the area who charge $300 per hour. Each chiropractor is well regarded but, as you can see, charges at a completely different rate.

How do you keep informed about the latest research and techniques for my condition?

Providers should tell you the journals they read, conferences they attend, as well as any classes they are taking.

Will you explain test results, as well as the risks and benefits of the recommended treatment?

Sometimes the provider will only share with you the test results he or she feels you should know. If you want all the results of tests, including reports, indicate that to the provider. Also, find out if there is a fee for your copy of the reports.

Do you consult with anyone for cases such as mine?

A secret among health care providers is that the provider is only as good as his or her resources. If this provider consults with a highly respected, superbly skilled health care provider who has vast experience healing your physical problem, you know that whatever arises, this provider will have access to a source who can really help.

Also, if this provider has a variety of health care professionals with whom he or she consults, that is a good indication that they have a good *network* of resources and that they are thorough in their care for their patients.

Who is on call when you are not available?

This is an important question — especially if your condition has the potential of escalating into a health care crisis that needs immediate attention. If you need immediate care from your health care provider and your provider is not available, you could get whoever is on call — a provider who may not have the skill or the bedside manner of the provider you've carefully chosen.

A friend of ours had a first-hand experience with an on-call provider. She was looking forward to the birth of her first child and was very pleased with the compassionate care she had received from the physician she had chosen. But when her labor began, her physician was on vacation. The physician who replaced him was more interested in getting back to his golf game than treating her competently. So he left her in labor for an unnecessary twenty-four hours before finally performing a cesarean section. Had she any idea that she would have received such terrible care from the doctor on call, she would have chosen her physician differently.

Making a Choice: Is This the One for You?

Now that you've completed your initial meeting with this provider, take a look at all the information you've gathered to make a decision about this professional. While reviewing the meeting, you may come to a quick decision as to whether this provider can work for you. It is more probable that you found both good and bad things about this provider.

To get some clarity as to whether you should cross this provider off your list or move forward with this provider, answer the following questions for yourself:

Has this person answered your questions adequately?

While you listened to the provider's answers to all your questions, did you have his or her full attention? Did this professional answer your questions completely and to your satisfaction? If not, that is red flag.

Author and medical educator Joan Borysenko, Ph.D., says, "A practitioner who doesn't adequately answer your questions has, in fact, given you valuable information — that you need to go elsewhere. Interview as many people as you need to; you don't have to feel obliged to make a return visit or even to carry our their recommendations."[8] If you didn't have the person's full attention during the interview or didn't get the answers you need, chances are you won't have the person's full attention or get the answers you need later on during treatment.

Did any of this person's answers raise concerns that are important to you?

Getting your questions answered gives you important information as to whether this is a health care professional you would want to work with. If important concerns were raised for you during the interview, you need to address those with the provider. If his or her responses to your concerns do not satisfy you, it would be best for you to continue to interview other providers on your candidate list.

Do you believe this health care professional has the skill and experience you need to reach your health care goals?

If you do not feel confident that he or she will give you the health care treatments you need and/or the quality of care you require, then it is best that you continue to look elsewhere.

Is this practitioner caring and compassionate enough for you?

If caring and compassion are important to you, do you believe this provider is the right personality type for you? It is true you may need to accept a competent provider with a less-than-compelling personality. But first see if you can find one who is both competent and compassionate, if that is important to you.

By answering these questions you will be able to know if this health care provider is a match. Even if you feel good about the provider, we encourage you to interview at least two other providers on your candidate list. You might find one you feel even better about!

If you have any doubts whatsoever about this health care professional, continue to interview other providers. Talk to as many providers as you need to make a clear and confident decision. Don't rush yourself. Invest the time to get quality care you want and deserve. Your health is worth it.

WHAT'S NEXT

By successfully doing Step Four, you have experienced firsthand some of the professionals on your candidate list. You got a feeling for who they are as a person as well as what they had to offer you professionally. More than likely you found at least one health care professional you can work with. Possibly you have even found several you feel good about, even though you have chosen the one you feel best about.

Now you are ready to move into Step Five: Form a Partnership. Step Five gives you the tools and the information you need to build a health care partnership between you and your provider. You will learn how to create an active alliance which will further support you in the healing process. By forming a health care partnership with your provider, you set up a situation that can both motivate and support, as well as educate and inspire you. 🖋

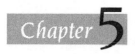

Chapter 5

STEP FIVE: FORM A PARTNERSHIP

A *Relationship You Can Live With*

The patient/physician relationship can become a sacred experience where each comes to trust and even love the other, and each learns and grows because of the other.

— David Hibbard, M.D. [1]

A health care professional as a "partner" may be a new concept for you. As a result, you may feel like you'll be making up the rules as you go along. For the most part, you will be. Given this, it is important to be open and flexible when forming this new kind of partnership with your health care provider. Keep in mind that your goal is to have a beneficial alliance with a health care professional so you can get healthy. Remember to keep the concept of getting healthy your main objective.

If you have done the first four steps as outlined in this book, by the time you get to this step you already know:

- The latest information on your health condition
- Some of the most effective treatments being used by health care practitioners around the world and how they may or may not apply to your condition
- The type of personality you need in your health care provider
- A health care provider you feel is competent and is a good "match" for you and your needs

With this information you have prepared yourself to form a good, workable health care partnership, one that will respect the knowledge you have gathered so far, which will be able to meet your needs as you journey together down the road to recovery.

Norman Cousins' Story: His Friend for Life

I first met Bill Hitzig socially — probably at some dinner. Then we became partners in various medical enterprises. When I organized a medical project to treat people of Hiroshima after the atomic bomb, I recruited him to be a part of it. We shared a good deal — even long before my illness. I became the godfather to some of his children, and I named one of my daughters after his wife. It was a very special professional and personal relationship.

When I was diagnosed with my illness [a life-threatening form of arthritis], I had several advantages: I had confidence in my doctor and also confidence in what the human body had to offer. In my studies, I realized that the overwhelming majority of illnesses are self-limiting. That enabled me to be free of the panic and the depression that so frequently affects and inflicts the patients who have just been diagnosed with a serious health problem. I've seen many times that panic and depression create a hothouse for rapid advance of the disease. I wanted to avoid that particular condition.

I also found over the years that doctors take their cues from the patient. If the patient has a serious illness and reflects it in his attitude and behavior, the doctor feels he or she is in an uphill situation, and sometimes flails around. So I tried not to terrify my doctor by alarming him about my problems. Reassuring my doctor gave him the opportunity to give me the most important thing I needed — reassurance too.

My doctor was a man of rare insight. He understood the person, not just the disease that might affect the person. Some doctors make a diagnosis and everything else becomes a matter of textbook procedure. I realize now how lucky I was to have a doctor who understood there were things that could be done for me apart from the prescription pad.

He had the ability to commit himself to his patients. He went the extra mile, sometimes quite literally. One time — in the middle of the night — he drove from New York all the way to my home in Connecticut. That's dedication.

Also, he wasn't too proud to listen or even to learn from his patients. Most patients would feel intimidated to express their own ideas about their physical condition, but he would draw you out. Consequently, I felt comfortable about making suggestions about my own treatment, which in retrospect turned out to be rather relevant.

I have a much keener appreciation for my doctor and the relationship we had now than at the time. It was a mutual trust that developed into a very deep friendship. [2]

WHAT YOU WILL LEARN IN THIS CHAPTER:
- *The four cornerstones to all good health care partnerships*
- *The four key "Points to Consider" in forming a good health care partnership*
- *The four action steps for forming a successful health-care partnership*

The Four Cornerstones to All Good Health Care Partnerships

All good health care partnerships are founded on the following four cornerstones:

1. Mutual respect and caring
2. Honest communication
3. A shared commitment to healing
4. A treatment contract

1. Mutual respect and caring

In the past two decades, scientific research has shown caring to be a powerful healing force. Caring can be expressed in many ways, but the one constant in all its various expressions is the human bond — a bond where people interact with mutual respect resulting in profound benefits to each other.

In the health care partnership, many times *both* partners benefit from the experience in the form of a healing on some level. For the health care provider, many have found emotional and spiritual healing from working with courageous and loving patients who have so moved and inspired them that they are forever changed.

Patients also benefit tremendously from the health care relationship. The scientific evidence indicates that when you create a partnership with a health care professional who you know cares about you, you actually respond better to their treatments.

The bonding that occurs in partnership is so powerful that some providers feel it is more important than the type of medicine practiced. Len Wisneski, M.D., medical director of the Marriott Corporation, is one of those providers. "I feel we all have our own healing process and that the human bond that we form with others in a caring situation is the most important additive to supporting the body to heal," Dr. Wisneski says. "What we do — even the techniques that we use — take a back seat sometimes to the power of caring." [3]

Unleash this bonding power in your health care partnership by bringing mutual respect and caring to your own health care experience. Here are some ways to encourage these feelings between you and your health care provider:

- Be considerate of each other's feelings: Recognize that your health care provider is a human being like you. Don't assume that holding the provider position doesn't have its stresses too. It is important to hold him or her to the high standard of care you want and at the same time appreciate the constraints he or she is operating under as a person and a professional.

- Listen with genuine interest: One of the most common break-downs of any relationship is the lack of good communication. A common source of that breakdown is that one or both parties aren't listening. If you have closed off your mind to particular recommendations and observations of your provider, you can be sure that healthy balanced communication will be missing in your partnership. Listen respectfully. This professional has spent untold hours of study and training to learn about how to help you. Make sure the provider knows you value his or her input.

- Agree to disagree, if necessary: It isn't critical that you and your health care provider always agree on all issues — including which treatments to use. The key is to be able to come up with a plan together that takes into consideration both of your concerns and recommendations. This may take some negotiating so that both of you feel you are doing your particular job competently, but the benefits are more than worth it.

  If you cannot come to agreement about treatment and you feel strongly that you want to try a particular approach that your provider cannot support, expect your provider to document his or her protest strongly in clinical notes in order to protect him- or herself professionally and legally. Also, your health care provider may want to bring an associate in to witness his or her interaction with you as well as to have you sign a disclaimer to further protect his or her practice.

- Respect each other's unique perspective: As a patient, you hold a valuable and worthy point of view about what is going on in your body and how you'd like to manage it. In truth, it is *your* body. However, your provider has an extraordinary amount of knowledge and information on how the human body works and how to help it heal. Because of this, your provider can probably be more objective about your physical condition than you. This perspective may help bring some calm and sanity into your recovery process.

2. Honest communication

Good two-way communication between you and your health care provider is essential and can smooth some of the rough edges present in most health care relationships today. The more open and honest you each are with one another, the better your chances of having an effective health care partnership despite the difficulties that can arise.

Stanley Krippner, Ph.D., author and professor at Saybrook Institute in San Francisco, agrees and adds, "I think it is very important for the patient and doctor to have good communication. If the channels are not clear, the patient will not tell the physician everything he/she needs to know, and will not listen carefully to any good advice the physician might give. It's very important for both members of this team to be heard. Each partner has a responsibility in the communication process if the health care partnership is to work effectively." [4]

Even if you think your provider won't like what you have to say, take a deep breath and courteously say it anyway. If the provider doesn't know that you have misgivings, or questions, or even an opposing viewpoint, those issues and questions will never be addressed. And your provider will think you are both in agreement when, in truth, you aren't. This type of miscommunication is a breeding ground for a malpractice case and even worse: you being physically injured. Avoid misunderstandings by stating your case firmly and professionally.

Also, your health care provider carries an important position as a communicator in this partnership. It can be a real asset to have a provider who can deliver grave news in a supportive and caring manner. For example, imagine that your doctor has just informed you that you have terminal cancer and that you have a one in five hundred chance of survival. Certainly that would be frightening news. However, if that same doctor said, "Listen, I have to tell you what the statistics say, but I know a few people who have beaten this thing. If they can, so can you!" That message would help you rally your courage to face this disease and fight for your life. Make sure that your provider knows that you'd prefer to be inspired rather than frightened by his or her information.

3. A shared commitment to healing

Each party in the health care partnership has certain duties and responsibilities. It is the commitment to perform these important duties with dedication that creates the opportunity for healing to occur.

Let's look at the patient's duties first:

Roman dramatist and statesman Seneca said two thousand years ago, "It is part of the cure to wish to be cured." According to today's experts, this ancient truth about healing is still true today. The most important choice a patient can bring to a health care provider/patient relationship is the wish to be truly helped by the professional and the wish to truly help oneself.

A commitment to your own healing may require you to make major changes in how you live your life. For example, you may have to change habits you've had for decades — what you eat, how you exercise, as well as certain beliefs and attitudes you hold about yourself and your world. If those changes are necessary, only you can make them. The provider can't do them for you. Are you willing to make the changes required to help your healing take place?

Some people aren't willing to help themselves. At Dr. Christiane Northrup's Women to Women clinic, she says she has had patients who exhibit "victim thinking" — who say they want help but have an internal emotional structure that says, "Help me. You can't." She says they won't ever let the provider really help because they won't help themselves.

You can avoid this particular trap by being willing to face yourself and your illness and have the courage to make the changes necessary for your return to health. Your job as the patient is to do whatever you need to do and change whatever you need to change to get healthy. Help *yourself* so that your provider can help you.

On the other hand, your health care provider has duties in this partnership, too. His or her job is to do whatever he or she needs to do to achieve the partnership's health care goals. This can take many forms:

- Using treatments and techniques in which the provider is well-trained and experienced.
- Being available to the patient for questions and/or appointments as needed.
- If necessary, researching other treatment options through colleagues and medical literature.
- Embracing a willingness to consider and review treatment options the patient may have found in his or her own research.
- Having a commitment to assist the patient find other treatment options and experts if the desired results are not achieved in a timely manner.

This can seem like a tall order for a provider to fill, but the good ones assume these duties anyway. Here's a good example:

Recently we had the pleasure of working with a chiropractor, Dr. Robin Mayfield, who assumed these duties of the health care partner with dedication and compassion. At the time we were beside ourselves with frustration. Our two-and-a-half-year-old son, John, had one sinus infection after another for an entire year. We tried everyone and everything we thought might work — including several rounds of antibiotics. Nothing was working. He was almost constantly in pain. He was emotionally spent and so were we.

Dr. Mayfield was very compassionate and sensitive to John at their first session. She used Applied Kinesiology to diagnose the source of his problem; as well as chiropractic, homeopathy, and nutritional supplements as treatments. Her diagnostic technique was so non-invasive and her touch so gentle and effective that John immediately found some relief and announced that he wanted to come back soon so that "Dr. Robin could 'fix' me again."

John went back to see "Dr. Robin" *several* times because the sinus infection, though greatly improved, still hadn't gone away. At one point, she said she had used all her tricks in her doctor's bag so she suggested we all (she, Michael, and Mary) keep our eyes and ears open for treatments we weren't currently aware of. We had heard from a friend that colloidal silver was helpful in handling some infections. Dr. Mayfield researched this treatment, and after she was satisfied that it could help, she tried it on John. Soon we saw some good results.

But the final piece of this frustrating puzzle turned out to be — of all things — the ventilation system in our house. Dr. Mayfield had suspected that John might be irritated by something inside our home. And sure enough, she was right. The previous owners had been heavy, heavy smokers. When Monster Vac — that's really the name of the company! — came to clean out our vent system, they found pounds and pounds of tiny dust particles laced with smoke. Once that dust was out of our house and — better still — out of John's respiratory system, he recovered. Now he's out of pain. He gets a full night's sleep and so do we!

Dr. Mayfield is a good example of a provider who works in partnership for several reasons. Other providers who examined John said, "Oh, kids this age always have respiratory problems," and left it at that. She knew, however, that something was *wrong* and continued to work in his behalf until the problem was solved. She also kept in close contact with us through returned phone calls and sessions at her office, if necessary. When she had reached her limit of treatment options, she honestly communicated that to us and suggested we get involved in the search. When Michael and I found another option, she checked it out without hesitation and after researching it was willing to try it. Finally, she trusted her instincts and suggested we check inside the house for possible irritations. The best part of Dr. Robin's participation in this six-month process was that she kept John's recovery a fixed goal — not her need to be right. Our son's health was always her primary focus.

Hold your provider to this high standard, and you may be amazed at what you can accomplish together!

4. A treatment contract

When you are forming a partnership with your provider, it's wise to have a written contract that spells out what the provider will do, what you as the patient are expected to do, agreed upon treatments, and the estimated time needed to reach your health goal.

Generally this agreement will center around a treatment program that your provider recommends or that you create together. If unforeseen changes occur during the course of treatment, either party can always initiate renegotiation of the terms. But having a contract keeps both partners clear about what is expected and keeps the focus on the desired results.

Before discussing the details of the partnership contract, let's first look at who is responsible for choosing the treatment. Most people don't realize this, but it is the *patient's* responsibility to choose the treatment. The provider's responsibility is to recommend treatment options based on his or her experience, expertise and research *and* to explain them to you in as much detail as you require.

Consumer Reports' The Savvy Patient states, "You have a right to decide, in effect, what you are willing to pay in discomfort, in personal risk, and in money to get the diagnostic information or the benefits of the proposed treatment . . . This right to choose rests on a presumption that you are competent — a legal, not a medical term. This means that you are in full possession of your mental facilities and can choose rationally. Bear in mind, if you forfeit the right to decide, the doctor [or health care provider] will almost certainly make the decision for you. Some of the decisions may be irrevocable and some may not be those you might have chosen to make . . . "[5]

This is not a responsibility to take lightly. Be sure — first and foremost — that you have all the necessary information about this treatment before you agree to it: its efficacy, side effects, length of needed treatment, and cost, to confidently agree to the provider's treatment plan. Because when you agree to treatment, you run the risk of the wasting precious time, particularly if the treatment is ineffective or injurious. Refer to Step One to gather pertinent information regarding any treatment recommended to you. In the end, it is you, the patient, who has to live with the treatment's results.

Some people wonder, though, how a provider will react to the *patient* deciding on the treatment. Won't the provider get angry? Some will, but good providers who *want* to be partners with their patients are very supportive of their patient claiming their right to choose. John Upledger, D.O., is founder and president of the Upledger Institute. His perspective is a good example of this open support. "The choices have to come from the patient," he says. "I like to give them my opinion of their options. But I want them to know that it is only my opinion. I want them to know that the choices are theirs. Especially I want them to know that whatever choices they make, if they want us to be with them, we will. We're not going to kick someone out — which so often happens — if they choose to integrate chemotherapy and surgery with whatever we happen to be doing. We don't have an investment in having it happen our way."[6]

Again, the treatment choice is yours, not the provider's. When you negotiate your treatment contract, you can make sure that both your provider and you are in agreement of that fact and how it will affect your decision-making process together.

Once you are confident in a treatment or treatment program, you can clarify *your* duties and responsibilities as well as the provider's by including the following points in your contract:

- The agreed-upon health care goals and the dates you hope to reach them
- How your questions and concerns will be answered
- If you can get an immediate appointment during an emergency
- How you will know if treatment is working and how soon that will be
- Any changes you should report to the provider
- If recommended treatment doesn't work, the "Plan B"
- If the provider will seriously consider treatment options you find
- Any lifestyle changes you need to make
- Ways to support the healing process in addition to the

treatment program

- At what time, and through the presence of what symptoms, will you both conclude that you as the patient need to seek help from another health care provider
- If that occurs, will the provider refer you to another professional or will you have find your own referrals

Farther in the chapter is the section, Four Action Steps for Forming a Successful Health Care Partnership. There you'll find the details for creating this partnership contract. With your contract in hand, both you and your provider will be confident in trusting the other to actively strive for the common goal, your health.

Four Key Points to Consider in Forming a Good Health Care Partnership

To make sure you form a successful partnership with your health care provider, there are four key points you need to keep in mind. If you know about them in advance, they won't take you by surprise and undermine your ability to create this special bond. These four points may seem obvious to you, still we encourage you to ponder them because they can greatly affect the outcome of your health care.

The four key points to consider in forming a good health care partnership are:

1. Your health care provider is a professional.
2. Your health condition can greatly influence the kind of partnership you are able to form.
3. A good health care partnership requires "give and take."
4. You can bring caring into your partnership — even if your partner seems incapable of caring for you.

1. Your health care provider is a professional.

You need to appreciate and respect the fact that your health care provider comes to your partnership with certain constraints already imposed by the fact he or she is the professional. Professional standards, codes of ethics, licensing requirements, as well as the ever-present threat of malpractice suits, can all influence the behavior and recommendations of your health care professional.

Author Larry Dossey, M.D., speaks to this point when he says, "A patient who expects to find a physician [or health care provider] who will let her/him call all the shots, including selecting all the tests, may find it a difficult thing to do because of the very real risks created for the doctor. If a physician did opt for this sort of partnership and did not defend his diagnosis or therapeutic plan with 'tests'; if he were later sued by the patient, he would not have a leg to stand on in court. Those are simply the facts, as abhorrent as they might be. So the decision to enter into a doctor-patient relationship of the 'shared responsibility' variety is extremely complex, and can be largely shaped by forces quite beyond the personal philosophy of the physician."[7]

2. Your health condition can greatly influence the kind of partnership you are able to form.

The nature of the partnership you form with your health care professional may be substantially determined by the nature of your health condition. If you're in a possible life and death situation in which immediate action is required, the conversations you have with your health care partner will probably be very short and to the point — with your partner essentially calling the shots. This could make your "partnership" appear very "one-sided" when it comes to shared decision making, and for good reason.

Providers who treat patients who are very, very sick and who ignore potential legal repercussions put themselves at great risk. Unfortunately many health care providers have lost their license because they 'went along' with the patient's intuitions. Many were later sued when things went wrong.

If you are in a risky health care crisis, it might be wise to give the reins of controls and power to the professional until you are able to participate as a more active partner. If you are dealing with strong emotions, great physical pain, and discomfort, or a life and death situation, you may not be in the right frame of mind to be an active partner in your own health care. Letting the doctor do his or her job and "run the show" in circumstances such as these may be the best choice you can make as a partner. Of course, it should be understood and included in your health care contract that your goal is to be a more participative partner once the crisis has past.

On the other hand, if your health care situation is not a life and death scenario, you probably have the freedom to form a very different kind of partnership with your health care provider where your thoughts, feelings, and suggestions become a very important dimension of the partnership. More give and take can occur in such a situation and the possibility of a jointly created treatment plan becomes more likely.

As you can see, the health care partnership can exist in a variety of forms. It can also change form as your condition changes. The key is to make sure you have a partnership that works for you and your provider — and that you both understand and have agreed on the terms of your partnership.

3. A good health care partnership requires "give and take."

Learning your options, getting good referrals, screening the candidates, interviewing the provider, and forming a partnership are all steps you can take to control much of your health care experience. However, at times, being willing to give up to the expert is the wisest action to take. If that moment comes, do it graciously. Dr. Northrup shares an example of someone who does this skillfully:

"One of my patients had Hodgkin's disease twice. She has always gotten fabulous medical care because of who she is, and somehow, she knows how to work within the [conventional] medical system in an empowered way. I see her doing this by being willing to take some responsibility for the treatment choices and *at the same time* being ready to release some of the control to the experts when it's necessary.

"When she starts her relationship with a health care provider, she says, 'Listen, I want to do the best I can for my body — and I don't want to be reckless. I'd like your expertise but I am ultimately responsible for my body. So whatever we do needs to feel right to me.'

"When her condition got a bit scary a while ago, here's what she did: She was in the hospital and her white blood count was very low from chemotherapy. Surrounding her bed were all the white-coated young doctors in training telling her she needed a transfusion. She said, 'Listen, guys, I know that's what you think, and that my blood count looks a little dangerous. But I feel I can get that blood count up if you give me three hours and a massage from *my* massage therapist here in the hospital. In three hours I want you to draw my blood again, and if I can't get my blood count up, then I'll go along with the transfusion.' The doctors said, 'No problem.' So she did some visualizations, and got a massage. And by the end of the three hours, her blood count was just fine." [8]

It is important that *both* partners are willing to "give and take" in order to achieve the goal of health for the client.

4. You can bring caring into your partnership — even if your partner seems incapable of caring for you.

If your health care partnership looks like it'll be lacking in caring because you had to pick a health professional who has little compassion, but, more importantly, has the necessary high skill level or special expertise you need, it's easy to shrug your shoulders and say, "Oh well, caring isn't available here." But don't let that stop you from creating what you want and/or need in any health care relationship — even if it's not obvious that you'll get it!

Author and surgeon Bernie Siegel, M.D., gave an example of how one woman changed her relationship with her M.D. She wrote to Dr. Siegel saying, "I had an appointment with my internist. To put it in a few words, I let him know how he made me feel: unloved and that I was taking up too much of his time. I told him that I wasn't *only* an intestine — that I had a mind and feelings too. Well, the long and short of it was, yes, I did let all my feelings out, but then we hugged each other. I called him 'Jay' (his first name) and told him I was hurting. We hugged and told each other that we loved each other. What a change from the cold machine I thought he was!" [9]

To get a provider who's also a partner, start with the provider right in front of you. Many times, when you really make the effort to verbalize your needs and make the provider see you as a human being, the provider responds. He or she will see you differently and therefore, will treat you differently.

Remember, health care providers are human beings just like you. Their pressures and responsibilities sometimes make it difficult to keep their emotions at the forefront. But a health care provider who is treated with compassion and caring many times *becomes* compassionate and caring.

The Four Action Steps for Forming a Successful Health Care Partnership

To make sure that you get the result you want from your health care partnership you must be an *active participant* — not just at the beginning but throughout the whole course of your treatment and recovery. You must be *proactive on your behalf* if you are to reach your health care goals.

There are four actions steps that will assist you in this process:

1. Be responsible for agreeing to, monitoring, and evaluating the treatments you receive.
2. Negotiate a "health care contract" with your provider.
3. Support your healing physically, emotionally, mentally, and spiritually.
4. Practice balancing flexibility with inflexibility.

1. Be responsible for agreeing to, monitoring, and evaluating the treatments you receive.

Again, being in a thriving health care partnership means that each party shoulders *his or her* responsibilities in the partnership. Just because you are in partnership with a health care professional doesn't mean that you relinquish your responsibility for choosing the treatments! Also, it is up to you *with your partner* to monitor and determine if the treatments are working for you as expected.

Once the professional has recommended a treatment, let the provider know how much time you'll need to make a choice.

If you don't have confidence in the treatment this provider recommends, ask what will you lose or gain by waiting. If you have the time, use the resources in Step One to get as much detail as you need to be certain about the treatment. *Consumer Reports' The Savvy Patient* states, "A patient who has just been informed that she has a lump in her breast, a spot on her lung, or an abnormal EEG is under tremendous pressure to do something, and to make a decision. As a result, such a patient is likely to accede to whatever course of action the doctor may recommend or — more likely — simply orders. The problem is that this is just the time for that patient to step back to reflect on the information, to gather more information, and to consider options and preferences. In most medical problems, a delay of a day or two will have no effect on the course of the disorder or the effectiveness of whatever treatment is chosen." [10]

Do what you need to do to be as sure as you can that this treatment is right for you before agreeing to it. Once you have decided, realize that it's not unusual for doubts to arise:

Helene Smith is a molecular biologist. As the director of the Geraldine Brush Cancer Research Institute at the California Pacific Medical Center in San Francisco, she's considered one of the foremost cancer researchers in the world. She also has breast cancer. Through her work she is constantly kept informed of which treatments for breast cancer are working and which are not.

She's a renowned expert and knows about being informed; however, even *she* has doubts about the treatment choices she makes.

"In the end, you collect all the information you can, and then you have to trust your inner voice," she says. "I don't know how other people do it; I only know how I do it. There are many tools: I use meditation a lot . . . I've just waited for the answer to come, and in the end, I just know. And then after I think I know, I get scared and say, 'You don't really know,' and then I say, 'Tsk, maybe I was wrong!' and then I run a whole lot of tapes [in my mind], and then I go back to the place where it says, 'I know.' And then, that's what I have to do. Maybe I'm wrong but that's also part of living, to accept responsibility for making a choice and doing it." [11]

Once you do start a treatment with your provider, do it 100 percent *and* keep evaluating your progress. Keep daily notes in a journal of any changes you think are a result of the treatment. That way, as the days go by, you'll see clearly how and if this treatment has affected you. That way you can evaluate the effectiveness of the treatment. Also, keep in communication with your provider about any changes you notice so that he or she can correct the dosage, or initiate a new treatment.

Be sure to ask your provider for a *time line* as to when you can expect to see results — and remember to stick to the time line. Author Joan Borysenko, Ph.D., says, "A difficult problem arises when ineffective treatment is offered in a cooperative partnership mode. For example, I have seen several patients who had received acupuncture treatments for depression. Their practitioners had been skilled, compassionate, and caring. But the method of treatment — acupuncture — though very effective for many conditions, is not usually successful in treating depression. Unfortunately because the quality of the relationship with the practitioner was so good, these patients continued too long in a treatment that clearly wasn't working for them. When choosing a treatment — no matter what treatment you are considering — it is important to ask your practitioner first for a projected time frame for healing and to seek another kind of treatment if improvement doesn't happen within that time." [12]

2. Negotiate a health care contract with your partner/provider.

As suggested before, it is very important that you create a written agreement with your partner/provider that includes what he or she is going to do, and what you are expected to do. Also include time periods to review whether a treatment is going according to plan. Be prepared to negotiate these terms by bringing a written agenda that includes a list of your concerns, your priorities, and questions so that you can be concise and clear in your communications.

Do not depend on your health care provider to suggest this. Many are not familiar with how to write one and some are uncomfortable with the idea. Still, most are willing to participate in such a contract if you are clear about your need to have one.

During your initial meeting your provider should tell you what your diagnosis is, what the prognosis is, and his or her treatment recommendations. If there is anything in this professional's communication that is unclear to you, get clarification now!

Next, agree to the desired outcomes and the time needed to reach those outcomes. Here are some suggestions:

- Share with the provider your health care goals for this partnership. Ask him or her if he or she would recommend any other goals for you.
- Find out if this provider can commit to these goals with you. If not, ask why.
- If the provider agrees with the goals, how long does he or she estimate it will take to reach them?
- How will you know if treatment is working and how soon should that be?
- At what time and in the presence of what symptoms will you both conclude that the provider can no longer help you?

To assist you in reaching the desired goals, find out what this provider is willing to do. Make sure you can count on this provider to be a partner *with* you. Many times that means the provider needs to share a valuable commodity: time. Here are some recommended questions:

- Will you answer my questions and concerns directly or will I be talking to your staff?
- Can I get an immediate appointment if I have an emergency?
- If the treatment isn't working, do you have a "Plan B"?
- Will you consider any treatment options I find in my own research?
- If I need to find another health care provider to work with, will you help me find the right one?

Next, discover what *you* can do to reach the health care goal. Here are more suggestions:

- Please explain what I need to do in this treatment process.
- Are there any lifestyle changes I need to make?
- Are there any other actions I can take to support my healing process?
- What changes should I report to you?
- How often should I come back to be examined?
- Is there anything else you recommend?

Take notes. Ask any other questions you think of. Based on your conversation, draw up the terms of the contract, go over it with the provider, and make an agreement you both can live with.

3. Support your healing physically, emotionally, mentally, and spiritually.

There is a great deal you can do outside the provider's office to support your own healing. For instance, you can create a healing support system among your friends, peers, and appropriate professionals. Here are key areas to focus on:

Physically: There are many sources of information on how to strengthen your body. Most of them recommend a low fat, high fiber diet; appropriate exercise; stress-reducing exercises, such as yoga and meditation; and a good night's sleep. Don't expect great results of your treatment if you're making choices that weaken your physical strength, like eating junk food, not exercising, and playing at all hours of the night. Be wise. Use your common sense and self-control to help your body be healthy.

Emotionally: Some health care providers are not skilled in helping their patients through the roller coaster of emotions that emerge during a health care crisis. Many aren't trained for it. If your provider can't help you with feelings you are having a hard time with or the confusions that baffle you, find a professional, a friend, a clergy member, or a support group who can.

Mentally: Thoughts produce chemicals that can hinder or help healing. Take Norman Cousins' advice: make an effort to develop situations and relationships that inspire joy, laughter, and happiness. You'll feel better and you'll help your healing along.

Spiritually: Many people have found great relief and comfort in releasing their fears and pain to a higher source. If this fits within your belief system, take advantage of this "higher" option in whatever religion, faith, church, or spiritual teaching that inspires you to get "above" your challenges.

Ron Webeck used these principles and returned to health when no one — not even the M.D's — thought he could. Dr. Pachuta wrote about Ron in the *Maryland Medical Journal* saying, "I met a man who was sent home to die in a few months with AIDS and progressive multifocal leukoencephalopathy (PML). He had dementia, was nearly blind, and could barely walk or talk."

Ron's Recovery Story

The first time I heard anyone talk about being a long-term survivor of AIDS I thought, 'This guy was one of the lucky ones. It could never happen to me.'

At the time I was bedridden and was suffering from the effects of the AIDS virus in my spinal fluid as well as a brain disease. Briefly put, it is a disease that progresses relentlessly to paralysis, blindness, coma, and then death. I was already paralyzed on the left side, and I was losing my vision. So I could never even think that I would become a long-term survivor. I don't recall what that man said because I was searching as to how to even begin!

Weeks passed before I realized that I had to make some choices. My first choice was to try — not only for myself but for those who love me. As those of us who get a diagnosis of AIDS know, we are not the only ones who have AIDS. The people who are around us and our family will be suffering with us.

So in my travel of getting better, I was doing what most of us talk about — eating well, getting rest. I continued to get better. It seemed almost a year had passed before my health lifted to the point where I trained myself to walk again by using walkers and canes.

It was about that time that I was fortunately pushed to a Louise Hay meeting in Key West. I had heard this theory of positive thinking and that it could help AIDS patients. I thought, 'This is ridiculous.' It just didn't seem true that anyone could recover just from a change in attitude.

But I went. A protégé of Louise Hay's talked about the benefits of positive thinking that helped him recover from cancer. It all started to make sense to me. I decided to try because I started to see love enter my life. For more than six months before [that moment] there was a lot of hatred and anger.

When I started to lift all that anger, there was some space for healing to begin. Then I started to do Uncle Bernie's [Dr. Bernie Siegel] work. One thing that struck me about cancer patients [in Bernie Siegel's book *Love, Medicine and Miracles*] is that they are recovering. If cancer patients and other people with so-called terminal illnesses can recover, why can't we?

As I was going into my second year of wellness or recovery, a lady friend of mine gave me a wonderful book called *Man's Search for Meaning*, written by Victor Frankl, a survivor of the Holocaust. It talks about how people in the concentration camp survived. It explains that everyone who survived had a common element between them. They had hope — hope that their lives would be liberated, and they would be free. It inspired me so much that I felt that maybe I was experiencing my own holocaust. Maybe AIDS was a holocaust of its own. After diagnosis we [people with AIDS] feel, 'What is there left to look forward to in life? We have AIDS. There's nothing more.'

But there is a greater question. What is life expecting from us? Maybe we have a commitment — to life, to others who will have AIDS — to make a prognosis of living long and living well.

In my public speaking many times they ask me, 'How did you get well?' As Frankl explains, it is not only the question of how you get well but why you get well. I chose to get well because I wanted to help other people and to make a difference. It is really the basic reason that has sustained my life for almost five years. [13]

4. Practice balancing flexibility with inflexibility.

When it comes to your personal health care, it can be especially baffling to determine when to be flexible and inflexible. Here are a few guidelines for your consideration:

- Be inflexible about treating your partner as you would like to be treated yourself.
- Be inflexible with yourself in shouldering the responsibilities you hold as the patient.
- Be inflexible about being compassionate with yourself in your current health crisis.
- Be flexible and open to the ideas and suggestions of your health care partner.
- Be flexible in your expectations about how and when your healing process is to occur. Sometimes the curative power of nature has its own timing.
- Be flexible with your habits and lifestyle so that it can serve your healing.

WHAT'S NEXT

By completing Step Five you join a growing number of health care consumers who have empowered themselves to take control of their health care destiny. Not only that, but by having completed all five steps you have learned how to be a more responsible health care consumer. You have gained the confidence that comes with becoming informed, as well as the self-respect that comes from knowing that you are choosing the treatments you receive in reaching your health care goals.

In the next section of this book you will take a journey into the terrain of alternative medicine. To prepare yourself for your journey, you will be given an overview of the thirty most popular alternative treatments as well as an in-depth, chapter-by-chapter look at the five major alternative health care systems that are licensed as primary health care providers in some or all areas of the United States.

PART II

❦

The Five Licensed Systems of Alternative Medicine

The Terrain of
Alternative Medicine

There is no prescription more valuable than knowledge.
— C. Everett Koop, M.D., U.S. Surgeon General [1]

By working through Part I of this book, you inevitably learned about a variety of alternative treatments that might help heal your health condition. In doing this, you might have found yourself becoming a little confused as you tried to understand exactly how and where those treatment options fit in the vast territory of alternative medicine. For this reason, having a good "map," or overview, of the alternative medicine terrain is essential to make sense of all these options.

To help you do this, you'll find a map of alternative medicine in this chapter. As you familiarize yourself with this overview, you will undoubtedly find it easier to make sense of all your treatment options and to determine which treatments might be right for you and your needs, as well as which health care providers can offer that treatment, or various treatments, to you.

Martin's Story: The Many Choices and Cures for the Common Cold

Two years ago, I went through what I now call the "year of the cold." Over and over, I kept getting this cold with flu-like symptoms that just would not go away and stay away. As a result of this ordeal, I had the opportunity to try a variety of different treatment approaches in my attempts to get better.

First, I went to my regular medical doctor, who offered me symptomatic relief by recommending over-the-counter medication, such as Tylenol, Advil, or Nuprin, to make me feel more comfortable. This particular M.D. was conservative with antibiotics and told me that since there wasn't an indication that my runny nose and congestion were bacterial in nature, he surmised that it was probably viral. Therefore, antibiotics wouldn't help me overcome this particular infection. In addition to the over-the-counter medications, my doctor recommended plenty of fluids and extra rest. While this helped me feel better, it did not permanently get rid of my symptoms.

At the suggestion of a good friend, I went to see a naturopathic doctor. She recommended more specific dietary changes than my M.D. did, such as avoiding dairy products because they can produce mucus (which I had plenty of already!), limiting sugars because they can create acids that can make a cold linger, and eliminating fats, which are even more difficult to digest when one is weakened with an infection.

She also offered other solutions to stimulate my immune system to fight off my cold. First she recommended fluids like diluted fruit juices, chicken broth, or miso garlic soup, and vitamin supplements of C, A, and Zinc. She also recommended a broad range of herbal treatments. Ginger tea would increase perspiration to help my body clean out toxins. Echinacea and golden seal tinctures both stimulate the immune system. Sage tea breaks up congestion and would bring down a fever (if it showed up). Eating garlic was also high on her suggested list, since it has antibacterial properties and would also help my body detoxify. I had read about the use of vitamin supplements for a cold in a health magazine I subscribe to, but this was the first time I had heard about these specific herbs and their healing properties. As I tried her recommendations, I found that my cold left and I had renewed energy and my thoughts were clearer. But about six weeks later, those same symptoms were back.

Out of curiosity, I decided to try another approach to healing my cold. The next health care expert I saw was a homeopath. She was an R.N. who had received further training at the British Institute of Homeopathy and College of Homeopathy. She asked me quite a few questions: how my throat felt, what was the color and consistency of my mucus, the foods I was craving, when I was thirsty, and how I was feeling emotionally. Based on my answers, she said my cold resembled the "profile" of Pulsatilla: stuffy nose with thick yellow discharge, worse at night and when indoors, the patient prefers to be outdoors and wants comfort and attention. She recommended six tablets of 30c Pulsatilla every one to two hours until my symptoms disappeared. She said homeopathic pills were easy to take because they tasted like sugar pills. However, they also have particular energetic properties. I thought, what a surprising way to diagnose and treat an infection.

The pills gave me some temporary relief. But, two days after I stopped taking them, my sniffles and stuffiness were back.

My neighbor suggested I try his chiropractor, who he swore could work miracles. The chiropractor said that my mid back and neck were out of alignment and he adjusted them by using a technique called spinal manipulation. My range of motion was much better in my neck after the adjustment, and despite my doubts that adjusting my neck could make much of a difference, I did feel somewhat better and had more energy. But, after a week, my sniffles were back.

An osteopath found that my cranial bones were causing some minor obstacles in the flow of my spinal fluid. After she gently adjusted my cranial bones, I was also pleasantly surprised by the results. My head felt less "muddy" and I could actually see a little more clearly. My sinuses began to drain like Niagara Falls! I felt I had finally found the answer, only to have my stuffiness come back three weeks later.

After reading an article about Chinese medicine, my final journey was to an acupuncturist who said that he could see immediately that I had an "unwanted guest" in my system. He placed his fingers on my wrist and took my "pulses." He asked me a few questions about how I was feeling, then asked to see my tongue. He nodded, and said that I had a "hidden fever" in my body that had been there for three seasons and that acupuncture could help my recovery. While lying on his massage table, he put some very slim needles in my upper back, one in each of my hands, and one in each of my ankles. I expected this to really hurt, but it didn't.

He left me there with the needles for about twenty minutes. When he returned, he had some Chinese herbs in the form of small pills that I was to take for the next two weeks to further my recovery. After he removed the needles, I definitely felt stronger — like the treatment had really helped me win part of the battle with this infection. I went back in two weeks for a follow-up treatment and some more pills. After this last treatment with the acupuncturist, my cold symptoms finally disappeared for good.

One thing I noticed about my adventure with all the alternative treatments is that my body felt stronger and better afterwards, even if the cold came back. Still, I think it was the combination of the acupuncture with the osteopathic treatments that finally helped me to overcome my "unwanted guest."

Looking back over the whole experience, I am still filled with wonder about all the different perspectives that healing professionals have to view and treat the same common cold. I have also come to realize that I have other treatment options besides over-the-counter drugs that can really make a difference in my overall health and well-being.

The Three Key Features on the Alternative Medicine Map

In looking at our map of the world of alternative medicine, there are three key features that stand out:

• First, we see *systems* of alternative medicine, much like a map of the world has countries.

• Second, we see that there are also *modalities* of alternative medicine, much like a map of a country would have states or provinces.

• Third, we see that there are alternative medical *treatments*, similar to the cities and towns within a particular state or province.

From our map we see that alternative medicine is made up of a rich variety of *treatments* (cities and towns), that fit into one of seven *modalities* (states or provinces), that are shared by eight major alternative medical *systems* (countries).

Systems of Alternative Medicine

How these modalities and treatments are combined is what gives each system of alternative medicine its uniqueness. It is this unique combination of modalities and treatments that makes each system of alternative medicine so special.

Just as all countries have certain things in common, all systems of medicine also have certain components in common, including:

• A definition of health and well-being

• An explanation for the cause and cure of illness

• Education and training of its providers

• Medical texts that describe the various treatments and remedies of that system

• Places where treatment is provided

• Laws and licensing requirements in most cases to assure high standards of treatment

• An underlying philosophy about reality, the meaning of life, what it means to be human, and a human being's place in the greater scheme of things

Each system of medicine has a history of growth and development as well as a core philosophy from which all diagnoses and treatment are derived. Most importantly, each system is based on a particular paradigm or view about what life is and how healing occurs. Often these beliefs are also unique to that system.

No one system of medicine is complete and perfect. All systems have certain illnesses and conditions they can treat effectively and also other illnesses and conditions for which they would not be the medicine of choice.

For example, the system of conventional biomedicine is considered the best in the world for emergency room trauma and epidemics. Yet, for chronic conditions, such as rheumatoid arthritis, it is not as effective. For chronic conditions, the systems of Chinese medicine, ayurvedic medicine, and naturopathic medicine have shown to be effective.

The eight of the more popular systems of alternative medicine are:

Ayurvedic Medicine is an ancient system of healing from India that treats the whole person with diet, nutrition, and lifestyle recommendations. The key components to this system of healing include the concept of "prana," or vital energy, the five elements (earth, water, fire, air, ether) and how well they are balanced in the individual, and the three constitutional types: vata, pitta, and kapha. The goal of Ayurveda is to bring about individual well-being so that spiritual development can take place.

Chiropractic is a system of health care that focuses on the relationship between the spinal column and the nervous system. By manipulating the skeletal system, nerve flow is increased to reduce pain and increase health. It is the treatment of choice for most cases of lower back pain. In the U.S., approximately one out of every ten Americans is under the care of a chiropractic doctor and 49 percent of all households in the U. S. have received chiropractic care. [2]

Environmental Medicine is a relatively new system of alternative medicine that studies and treats the impact of environmental factors on health and is based upon the concept that many illnesses are, at least partially, caused by our allergic reactions to the toxins in our modern-day environment. The effect of chemicals, foods, and the quality of the air one breathes are all evaluated to determine their effect on one's health. Herbs, large doses of vitamins and minerals, nutrition, and other treatments are used to clear toxins from the body and to restore health.

Ethno-Medicine/Shamanism/Native American Medicine — Throughout history all indigenous peoples around the world have developed ways to treat and heal their illnesses. Almost all focus on helping the patient discover the meaning of their illness for, in understanding the meaning, the remedy for their recovery is revealed. Many of these systems of healing use herbal remedies, Powwowing (counseling with a wise woman of the tribe), spiritual practices, and hands-on healing to achieve the recovery of health, and are still effectively used today. Shamans still practice among many tribes in Mexico as well as in Central and South America. In the United States such traditions are still carried on by the Lakota Sioux and Dineh/Navaho Tribes.

Homeopathy is a system of medicine that is almost three hundred years old and has been practiced in the U.S. since 1825. It is based on the "Law of Similars" that states that "like cures like." For example, a minute dose of belladonna, normally a poison in larger quantities, may be prescribed for symptoms that are similar to those of belladonna poisoning. Remedies for treatments are made from plants, animals, and minerals. It is believed that the minute nature of the doses stimulates a healing response in the body. The official remedy book *Homeopathic Pharmacopoeia of the United States* is recognized by the FDA.

Naturopathic Medicine is a system of medicine that utilizes natural therapies to stimulate the body's innate healing ability. The goal of all treatments is to raise the vital energy so that the body can reestablish health. It is rooted in the concepts of the healing power of nature, treatment of the whole person, doing no harm, and treating the cause. Built on treatments sometimes thousands of years old, it first gained great popularity in the U.S. in the 1920s.

Osteopathic Medicine was developed in the U.S. after the Civil War by Andrew Still, a surgeon who had served in the Union Army. It focuses on the relationship of body structure to organ function. One of its basic tenets is that structure and function are two sides of the same coin. For example, the integrity of the spinal column (structure) has a direct impact on nerve innervation to various organ systems in the body (function). For this reason, the skeletal muscular system is a key area of treatment for reestablishing health.

Traditional Chinese Medicine is one of the oldest systems of medicine in practice in the world today. The primary focus is on prevention and a natural view of the world with the person being a microcosm of that world. Also important is the concept of "chi," or vital force, and how well it is flowing and balanced in terms of the "yin" (feminine/receptive) and "yang" (masculine/assertive) principles of Chinese thought. Acupuncture, Chinese herbs, massage, food therapy, exercise, and lifestyle changes are some of the treatment methods used in this system. It is estimated that between nine and twelve million Americans receive Chinese medical treatments in the United States per year.[3]

Modalities of Alternative Medicine

As stated earlier, each system of health care draws on a number of modalities much like a country is made up of a number of states or provinces. For example, the modalities of surgery and pharmacology (drugs) and the various treatments associated with those modalities, are important components of the conventional biomedical system of medicine. On the other hand, in the system of Chinese medicine, the modalities of somatic therapies, herbal medicine, mind/body interventions, and the various treatments associated with those modalities are important components of that system.

A modality can be seen as the area of focus or specialty that the practitioner uses in order to diagnose or treat. Within a particular modality there can be a range of treatments or diagnostic techniques.

The seven major modalities of alternative medicine include:

Bioelectromagnetic Applications focus on both the positive and negative effects that various forms of electromagnetic energy have on our health. This includes the effects that electromagnetic fields (EMFs) from power lines and other sources, such as electric blankets and household appliances, have in causing leukemia, cancer, and a variety of immunosuppressant illnesses. The application of various forms of bioelectromagnetic energies are used in the treatment of osteoarthritis, bone repair, nerve stimulation, wound healing, immune system stimulation, and tissue regeneration. Treatments used include transcutaneous electrical nerve stimulation (TENS), cranial electrical stimulation (CES), photostimulation, magnetic field therapy, and electroacupuncture.

This modality is a key component of traditional Chinese medicine, environmental medicine, and osteopathic medicine.

Diet and Nutrition, as an alternative modality, is used for the prevention and treatment of chronic disease. The goal is to counteract the negative health consequences of the modern affluent diet. The advent of processed foods, fast foods, additives, preservatives, hydrogenated oils, coupled with the removal of whole grains, fruits, and vegetables from the American diet have had a damaging effect on the health of many people. Such diet and nutritional techniques as macrobiotics, Gerson Therapy, orthomolecular medicine (megavitamin), lifestyle changes, nutriceuticals, fasting, vitamins and mineral supplements, raw juice therapy, Kelly regimen, Ornish Diet, Pritikin Diet, Wigmore treatment, Livingston/Wheeler regimen, food elimination for treatment of food allergies, Mediterranean Diet, and vegetarian diets all have claims to help heal certain health conditions.

Diet and nutrition can play a major role in ayurvedic medicine, chiropractic, environmental medicine, naturopathic medicine, osteopathic medicine, and traditional Chinese medicine.

Energy Medicine involves the use of nonlocal, nonmeasurable energy sources. Many of these energies are still not accepted by mainstream science as existing since they challenge many accepted scientific paradigms. It can involve the measurement of subtle energy fields in and around the body that are used to determine the degree of illness and health. Homeopathy, psychic healing, spiritual healing, prayer therapy, radionics, flower essences, acupuncture, and certain shamanistic practices are some of the treatment techniques used.

The modality of energy medicine is important to the following alternative medical systems: ayurvedic medicine, ethnomedicine/shamanism/Native American medicine, homeopathic medicine, naturopathic medicine, and traditional Chinese medicine.

Herbology/Phytotherapy are any interventions that utilize herbs and botanicals. Evidence shows that this alternative modality was in use over sixty thousand years ago by our early ancestors. Its treatments are still effective today and are growing in popularity. [4] Many herbal products once only found in the old time pharmacy are now once again finding their way back to our modern store shelves. Some of the more popular herbs being used today include ginkgo biloba for Alzheimer's Disease, hawthorn berry extract for heart disease, valerian root extract for insomnia and anxiety, milk thistle extract for hepatitis, and saw palmetto extract for prostate problems. In fact, in Europe many doctors trained in conventional medicine freely prescribe these herbs under the heading of phytotherapy.[5]

This modality is a major component of the following alternative medical systems: ayurvedic medicine, environmental medicine, ethno-medicine/shamanism/Native American medicine, naturopathic medicine, and traditional Chinese medicine.

Mind/Body Interventions include those interventions that emphasize the profound interconnectedness between the mind and body and the influence each has on the other. Treatments such as guided imagery and active visualization, biofeedback, meditation techniques, relaxation techniques, hypnotherapy, art therapy, sound and music therapy, hatha yoga, t'ai chi, qigong, martial arts, dance/movement therapy, color and light therapy, and aromatherapy are just some of the more popular alternative mind/body treatments. Also included in mind/body interventions are all the various exercise programs designed to increase cardiovascular health, lymphatic flow, range of motion, and increased vital energy.

The mind/body modality is a major component of the following systems: ayurvedic medicine, ethno-medicine/shamanism/Native American medicine, naturopathic medicine, and traditional Chinese medicine.

Pharmacological and Biological Modalities are techniques that use substances that generally focus on stimulating the immune system as well as detoxifying the body. Some of these are in wide use, although they are still experimental in nature. None are approved by the FDA at this time, though many are prescribed and used freely in other countries. For these reasons many are quite controversial. Alternative medical treatments which are a part of this modality include anti-oxidant therapies (high doses of Vitamin E and Beta-Carotene to scavenge free radicals), ozone therapy for AIDS, chelation therapy for cardiovascular disease, metabolic therapies (shark cartilage, Naessens [714-X], Essiac, Hoxsey, and Revici), and cell treatments (Antineoplastons, Immunoaugmentation, MTH-68), apitherapy (bee venom), neural therapy for chronic pain, and Iscador (mistletoe) for immune stimulation.

This modality is not a principle component of any of the major alternative medical systems, though it may be used most often in environmental medicine, naturopathic medicine, as well as experimental biomedicine.

Somatic Therapies/Manual Healing includes those techniques that focus on touch and manipulation with the practitioner's hands on the physical body of the patient. They include such techniques as massage (Swedish, sports, Esalen, deep tissue, St. Johns, etc.), Rolfing, structural integration, Aston Patterning, chiropractic adjustments, osteopathic adjustments, Alexander Technique, Trager Method, reflexology, acupressure, craniosacral therapy, Feldenkrais Method, Hellerwork, Hakomi, Jin Shin Do, manual lymphatic drainage, postural integration, physical therapy, shiatsu and trigger point therapy.

This modality is a major component of ayurvedic medicine, chiropractic medicine, ethno-medicine/shamanism/Native American medicine, naturopathic medicine, osteopathic medicine, and traditional Chinese medicine.

Alternative Medical Treatments

As we mentioned above, just as each state or province is made up of cities and towns, so is each modality of alternative medicine made up of a rich variety of treatments. Treatments are the specific actions the health practitioner does to you or prescribes for you to support your healing/recovery process. Your practitioner may use only one treatment or several treatments that complement one another, based on your diagnosis and needs. If you are receiving more than one type of treatment, it is possible that the treatments are from different modalities or even different systems of medicine. For example, a naturopathic physician might treat you with an herbal treatment, such as feverfew, from the modality of herbal medicine and also prescribe a homeopathic treatment of Arnica from the medical system of homeopathy.

Some examples of the more popular treatments you might

encounter in your alternative medical journey include:

Acupuncture, as a treatment, is the insertion of a very fine needle into one or more of over one thousand acupuncture points located along twelve energy channels or meridians on the body. This treatment affects the flow of energy, which the Chinese call "chi," to help heal the patient. Acupuncture has been shown to be an effective treatment for pain, migraines, addictions, duodenal ulcers, tennis elbow, paralysis from stroke, osteoarthritis, as well as ninety-seven other conditions identified by the World Health Organization. [6]

Acupressure Massage is a style of bodywork founded on the same theory as acupuncture. In acupressure massage, pressure is placed on acupuncture points on the client's body with the therapist's finger-tip, knuckle, or an instrument called a "tei shin." It is intended to stimulate and balance the chi to help heal the client. Acupressure massage has been shown to be effective for muscular pain, headaches (including migraine), backaches, insomnia, gynecological problems, and gastrointestinal disorders. [7]

Aromatherapy involves the therapeutic use of essential oils for physiological and/or psychological healing through absorption by the skin or by inhalation. When properly used, essential oils have been documented to help such conditions as arthritis, circulatory problems, muscular aches, digestive upsets, menstrual problems, stress, as well as many emotional and mental problems. [8]

Biofeedback Training teaches patients how to regulate autonomic functions such as heart rate, pulse rate, and blood pressure by hooking them up to a biofeedback machine that tells them how and where they are holding tension. With this information a person can be taught how to determine when and where they are holding stress and learn how to relax. Biofeedback is used to treat such problems as migraine headaches, and stomach and intestinal disorders. [9]

Chelation Therapy is a painless, nonsurgical medical technique that removes unhealthy heavy metals from the body. The patient is given an intravenous drip of ethylene diamine tetraacetic acid (EDTA), a chelating agent that attaches itself to metal molecules and creates a new compound that is then excreted through the kidneys. Often practitioners recommend chelation therapy for people with diabetes, osteoporosis, heavy metal poisoning, atherosclerosis, arteriosclerosis, Parkinson's disease, and hypertension. [10]

Colon Therapy cleanses and detoxifies the large intestine by washing away collected fecal matter. This is done by douching the colon with lightly pressured water. Used mostly by naturopaths, this technique aids digestion and elimination by detoxifying the system. Colon therapy has been used to treat arthritis, digestive disorders, high blood pressure, and heart disease. [11]

Color/Light Therapy is as old as ancient Egypt and is used to enhance the physical, emotional, and spiritual aspects of the human body. Healing systems, particularly ayurvedic, have noted for centuries that color wields physiological and psychological influence on patients. Practitioners treat their patients with color in a variety of ways, including colored light, colored eye glasses, liquids contained in colored glass, wearing colored clothing, or eating colored foods. [12] In ayurvedic medicine, color is used to balance the mind, body, and consciousness. Other practitioners use it for motivation, relaxation, strengthening the specific organs that correspond with particular colors, to assist the body's innate healing capabilities, and to restore well-being. [13]

Craniosacral Therapy is a gentle manual manipulation technique that recognizes and remedies imbalances in the craniosacral system. This system is made up of the brain, spinal cord, cerebrospinal fluid, cranial dural membrane, cranial bones, and sacrum. According to *Alternative Healing: The Complete Guide to 160 Different Alternative Therapies* (Halcyon Publishing, 1993), "It is believed that within the craniosacral system, the brain expands and contracts as a means of transporting cerebrospinal fluid throughout the brain and spine. Through this mechanism of pumping and draining, nerve cells continually receive a fresh supply of nutrients to keep them healthy, similar to the way muscles receive nutrients via the bloodstream."[14] Practitioners of craniosacral therapies gently palpate the cranial bones to determine if any bones are creating obstacles in the normal flow of cerebrospinal fluid. By subtly adjusting the bony structures of this system, a practitioner reestablishes the healthy flow of this intricate system. Craniosacral therapy is used to treat headaches, head or neck injuries, ear and eye problems, dyslexia, hyperactivity, as well as to release trauma.[15]

Dance/Movement Therapy uses dance and movement of the physical body, as the vehicle to help clients experience their feelings through the sensation of physical movement. This technique seeks to assist the client to reclaim self-esteem, to restore a sense of individual identity, and to enhance or reestablish the synthesis of body and mind. Dance therapy treats many conditions, including physical disability, substance abuse, autism, geriatric-related difficulties, and loss of self-esteem for people confined to bed or a wheelchair.[16]

Fasting has been used since ancient times by the Romans, Greeks, Egyptians, and Chinese as a way of cleansing the body of deadly toxins and rebuilding vitality. Fasting can range from only drinking water to the use of raw vegetable and fruit juices to stimulate cleansing and healing of specific areas of the body. Many conditions such as eczema, psoriasis, rheumatoid arthritis, chronic headaches, bronchial asthma, and schizophrenia have all shown results with fasting.[17]

Flower Essences are made from "potantized" flowers, which act as catalysts to relieve the causes of stress. Specific remedies correspond with personality types or kinds of emotional/mental stress. Patients put drops of the remedy under their tongue several times a day until the desired result is accomplished. Flower essences have been shown to be an effective treatment for grief, stress, and other forms of emotional and mental trauma.[18]

Herbal Treatments were discovered over time by early medicine men and women through watching animals eat specific plants when they were ill as well as by trial and error. The centuries of our ancestors "watching and trying" have brought modern humans a cornucopia of potent and effective treatments for ailments and illnesses of all kinds. Modern medicine has taken advantage of many of the ancient herbal treatments and processed them into what we now know as drugs. Herbs can be administered in a variety of ways: as a hot tea, tincture, poultice, or herbal wine; or in capsules or tablets, syrup, ointment, or paste. Herbs generally originate in natural forms as plants but must be administered as a drug and used in the required dosage at the appropriate time to avoid unpleasant and hazardous results. Herbs have been used to treat a wide range of health conditions, including digestive problems, memory loss, heart conditions, prostrate problems, fevers, and infections.[19]

Humor Therapy has been shown to be a powerful treatment in helping the body heal.[20] Through the release of endorphins, which produce feelings of euphoria and well-being, the body's natural healing mechanisms are stimulated and healing is facilitated. Norman Cousins used humor therapy to heal himself of a life-threatening illness, which he documented in his famous book, *Anatomy of an Illness* (Bantam, 1979).

Imagery and Visualization techniques use images and feelings created in the imagination to focus the mind so that physiological changes occur. These techniques are successfully used in helping stress-related or life-threatening illnesses, as well as enhancing sports performances.[21]

Jin Shin Do is a bodywork technique that moves stagnant energy through the body by touching certain Japanese acupuncture points and using breathing methods. Its primary focus is to relieve pain, as well as physical and emotional tension.

Meditation and Relaxation Techniques have been used throughout the world for centuries. Several types exist. In the most common form, the meditator sits upright and focuses the mind on an object, sound, or word. There are physiological as well as emotional and spiritual benefits, for meditation has a calming effect on its users. Also, scientific evidence indicates that it can reduce high blood pressure, pain, and stress. [22]

Macrobiotic practitioners theorize that foods can enhance a person's perception of themselves and their lives as well as improve health. Although macrobiotics, per se, does not promote the eating of certain kinds of foods, most diets associated with macrobiotics include whole grains, miso soups, vegetables, and beans. They discourage eating meats, dairy products, refined sugars, and coffee. Macrobiotic lifestyle and diet have been successfully used to treat several forms of cancer. [23]

Magnetic Therapy (Bio Magnetic Therapy) has been used throughout history and uses the placement of magnets on the body or magnetic field(s) around the body to help heal or strengthen health. [24] Its beneficial effects have been proven by a study at the Massachusetts Institute of Technology, which found that magnets placed on the body increased blood flow and healing. Magnetic therapy is used to treat insomnia, to speed up the healing of wounds, to facilitate bone netting in broken bones that do not heal, and for arthritis.

One nursing mother we know was having trouble with her breast milk drying up. Her acupuncturist, who used various forms of energy medicine as his basis for healing, adhered small magnets around her breast in order to draw the energy back into that area. Within twenty-four hours, she began to have more breast-milk, which increased over the course of a week. She returned for weekly visits to have the small magnets replaced, and continued to breastfeed for another six months.

Nutritional Supplements are used in most alternative medical systems. They are tablets, powders, or liquids containing vitamins, minerals, amino acids, enzymes, as well as other nutritional factors. Their ingestion is intended to replenish the body of nutrients that have been depleted for many reasons, including stress, bad dietary habits, and/or aging. Replacing these essential building blocks of the body gives it the materials it needs to rebuild and heal naturally.

Orthomolecular/Megavitamin Therapy are treatments for disease in which patients are given nutrient supplements to correct imbalances or to replace depleted nutrients of the body. It is based on the concept that disease, mental or physical, can be traced to nutrient imbalances. Schizophrenia, depression, substance abuse, allergies, and hyperactivity are some of the conditions treated with orthomolecular therapy. [25]

Oxygen Therapy (also called Ozone Therapy) uses medically pure-grade ozone or triatomic oxygen (three atoms of oxygen) to kill bacteria, virus, yeast, and parasites and to treat ailments, including AIDS and cancer. [26] During oxygen therapy, correct concentrations of ozone are introduced to the body by enema, injection under the skin into the muscle, or by intravenous infusion (IV).

Polarity Therapy is a system of balancing the life force energy (i.e., prana, chi) of the body by the practitioner's use of his or her hands to direct and correct the flow of that energy in and around the body, as well as to stimulate pressure points, and to increase joint movement. Diet, exercise, and self-awareness processes are also included in a complete polarity therapy program. Polarity therapy has successfully been used to treat headaches, tension, and stress by promoting relaxation and renewed vitality. [27]

Prayer Therapy has been used by many religions around the world for centuries as a means to promote healing. Only recently has prayer therapy gained respect among the scientific community as research studies prove that prayer can effect the healing process.[28] As a result, it is now being used as an adjunct to conventional medical treatment in some complementary medical programs and in several major hospitals.[29] Two excellent books on the subject are *Healing Words: The Power of Prayer and the Practice of Medicine* (HarperCollins, 1993) and *Prayer Is Good Medicine* (HarperCollins, 1996) by Larry Dossey, M.D.

Reflexology is a form of bodywork based on the theory that the soles of the feet and palms of the hands are mirrors of the entire body and that every area of the body corresponds to a specific place on the hands or soles of the feet. The only instruments used in reflexology are the hands, which apply steady pressure to the appropriate point on either the hands or the feet. By stimulating these points, a reflex action to the corresponding part of the body is created, increasing nerve flow to that area. Reflexology does not treat illnesses, per se, but practitioners believe that stimulation can positively affect the body and its ability to heal. For this reason, it is used as an adjunct for many physical conditions, including digestive problems, menstrual difficulties, hypertension, and migraines.

Shiatsu literally means "finger pressure" in Japanese and refers to the Japanese version of acupressure. Practitioners perform a "hara" diagnosis by palpating the patient's abdomen and other areas. Once a diagnosis is determined, the practitioner uses fingers, knuckles, elbows, knees, and other body parts to apply varying degrees of pressure on some of the 660 trigger points of the shiatsu zones. Shiatsu is used to treat many problems, including deep tissue and bone bruises, as well as arthritis pain and migraine headaches.[30]

Soft Tissue Manipulation is a style of body work or massage that manipulates muscles and the connective tissue that surrounds them, called facia, and its intention is to realign the body segments. Practitioners use fingers, palms, fists, and elbows to balance the body so that it is in vertical alignment with gravity.

Benefits can include physical pain reduction, better posture and range of motion, as well as emotional trauma releases. Styles of soft tissue manipulation include Rolfing, Hellerwork, Aston Patterning, and structural integration.

Sound/Music Therapy involves playing or listening to music and seeks to improve, rejuvenate, or preserve a client's health. Music therapy is helpful for mental and emotional disabilities, substance abuse, sensory impairment, and learning disabilities.[31] It also supports self-esteem and personal insight while serving as a catalyst for the expression of emotions and feelings.

T'ai Chi/Qigong are mind/body exercises that increase and harmonize the flow of chi or vital energy force. The main components of t'ai chi and qigong are management of the physical body (posture), in conjunction with stilling of the mind and control of the breath. The most common exercises are the inward training exercise, the relaxing exercise, and the strengthening exercise. Qigong and t'ai chi help stimulate digestion and help to heal stomach and duodenal ulcers, constipation, and high blood pressure. Practitioners of these exercises experience decreased heart rate, enhanced respiration, and increased oxygen assimilation.[32]

Therapeutic Touch is a method of hands-on healing in which the practitioner centers him- or herself, then runs his or her hands lightly over the client's body while attuning themselves to any energetic disruption they might feel. If a practitioner feels a sensation of heat, cold, tingling, pulsation, electric shock, or tightness in a specific area, the practitioner then "sends" energy to that part of the client's body to help balance or heal that area. Two documented benefits of therapeutic touch are relaxation and pain reduction.[33]

Yoga literally translated, means "union." The practice of yoga seeks to unite body, mind, and spirit in a balanced manner through the use of "asanas," or postures, diet and nutrition, meditation, regulated breathing, and relaxation. There are many types or paths of yoga. However, hatha yoga (meaning "force") is probably the most well-known style that specifically focuses on physical health. Yoga enhances physical fitness and vitality while also strengthening body functions, such as circulation, elimination, respiration, and digestion.

Sharing and Borrowing in Alternative Medical Practices

In alternative medicine, sharing between systems, modalities, and treatments occurs quite often. For example, a naturopathic doctor may also be trained and certified in Chinese medicine as well as homeopathic medicine. A chiropractic doctor educated and licensed to primarily do chiropractic manipulations may also be trained and certified in biofeedback and herbology.

So, alternative practitioners trained originally in one system as their primary focus will many times also be trained in other alternative medical systems with their corresponding modalities and treatments — all of which may not be directly related to their original education or training related to their license! Because of this practice, it is extremely important to make sure that the alternative health care provider is well trained and certified in any adjunct systems of medicine, modalities, or treatments that are not a part of their primary credentials or license.

Here's an example how this may affect you as you try alternative medical providers. We have a friend who went to see a chiropractor who, in addition to providing treatments of chiropractic medicine, also claimed to be trained in acupuncture. She felt confident that she would get good quality care from this health care provider because he was a licensed practitioner. When she arrived in his treatment room, she explained to the doctor that her left hand was aching. She shared with him that she was concerned that she might be getting arthritis and had heard that acupuncture helps to relieve the pain. The chiropractor agreed and offered to give her an acupuncture treatment.

He told her to lay back on the treatment table, which she did.

Then he brought out an instrument that looked like a gun. She asked him what it was. He said it was a staple gun and that he was going to put a few staples in her hand. She was quite surprised at this because she had been previously treated with acupuncture for another physical complaint and staple guns were not a part of any Chinese medicine that she had ever heard of. She told us later, "I don't think I've ever moved so fast in my life. I was getting out of that room and out of that office as fast as I could." Later she checked to see just where the chiropractor had received his training to give acupuncture and she found out it was in a one-weekend course he had taken.

"There's no telling what this man was about to do to me!" she said. Needless to say, before making another appointment with a health care provider who offered acupuncture, she made sure the provider was well trained in Chinese medicine, which in most states requires at least three years of training and passing a rigid exam on acupuncture, not a one-weekend course.

By thoroughly doing Step Three and Step Four of this book, you can feel confident that any treatments you receive are from a practitioner who is adequately trained. Consider the story of a friend of ours who did just that. Elizabeth had given birth to two beautiful babies in two years. As a result, she developed a very bad case of hemorrhoids. When her chiropractor offered to treat her with acupuncture for this condition she was hesitant at first. Elizabeth trusted this practitioner as a chiropractor but was not sure if he was adequately trained to competently treat her with acupuncture. Upon questioning her doctor, she found he had also formally trained in a two-year acupuncture program and had passed an exam, giving him a Diplomate in Acupuncture. Given his credentials and a certain comfort level she had obtained by asking the right questions and hearing answers she liked, Elizabeth decided to try the recommended acupuncture treatments. As a result, after three treatments over a period of three weeks, her hemorrhoids went away.

As you journey into the terrain of alternative medicine, you need to make sure that your alternative practitioner is well trained in any specific treatments he or she wants to perform that are not a part of his or her original training.

WHAT'S NEXT

Now that you have an overview of the terrain of alternative medicine, the succeeding chapters will give you valuable details about the five systems of alternative medicine whose providers are licensed to offer general health care in the United States. They are the M.D. as an alternative practitioner, traditional Chinese medicine, chiropractic, naturopathic medicine, and osteopathic medicine.

Each chapter will address:

- Important facts about this system of alternative medicine
- Major medical treatments
- The health conditions that respond best to this alternative medicine
- Important points to consider before receiving treatment, specific information and actions to add to Steps One through Five, as well as key questions to ask before receiving treatment
- What to expect during an appointment, including costs, length of an average appointment, and general techniques
- Insurance information
- Education, training, and licensing requirements of the practitioner

Over the course of the next five chapters, you will have an opportunity to further your understanding of alternative medicine. Each chapter provides an in-depth look at one of the five major alternative medical systems and its licensed health care providers. This information, coupled with the Five Steps from Part I of this book, gives you all you need to know to competently begin your journey into the world of alternative medicine. As you do that, the chances are very high that you will find the right alternative treatment and the right practitioner to meet your own and your family's health care needs.

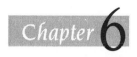

Chapter 6

THE M.D. AS AN
ALTERNATIVE PRACTIONER

Blending the Best of All Medicines

The village doctor was a great success. His success was due to his sympathy with his patients, each of whom he treated as an individual with an idiosyncrasy of his own and worthy of special and separate consideration. It was as if, instead of giving everyone mass-produced medicine, he had molded the portrait of each on his pill.

— Oliver St. John Gregory

DID YOU KNOW THAT:

- In the future, it is expected that the greatest number of practitioners of alternative medicine will be M.D.'s. [1]

- A recent survey of family physicians in the U.S. found that more than half regularly prescribe alternative treatments or have tried alternative therapies themselves. [2]

- In Resolution 514, the American Medical Association (AMA) "is encouraging its members to become better informed regarding alternative medicine and to participate in appropriate studies of it." [3]

- At this writing, thirty-seven or almost one-third of conventional medical schools, including Harvard, Yale, and Johns Hopkins, offer courses in alternative medicine. [4]

- Columbia-Presbyterian Medical Center in New York is one of a growing number of hospitals creating alternative medical clinics on site.

• Dean Ornish, M.D., developed a program that reverses heart disease, a feat previously considered impossible by the conventional medical community. All treatments in Dr. Ornish's program are considered alternative. [5]

An ever-increasing number of medical doctors are showing a genuine interest in practicing alternative medicine. [6] Many of them have come to appreciate that the American health care consumers who use alternative medicine may know something they don't about getting well. Many physicians are recognizing that they can be even better doctors for their patients by integrating unconventional and alternative medical treatments into their conventional practices. Because of this change in the opinions of M.D.'s about alternative medicine, many well-respected medical schools are now offering courses and programs in alternative medicine.

The Techniques of Alternative Medicine vs. the Spirit of Holistic Medicine

The idea of medical doctors becoming even better doctors for their patients is very good news because conventionally trained M.D.'s are skilled experts in a valuable system of medicine. Add to this expertise in conventional medicine a commitment to compassionately serve the patient as a person, plus an expertise in effective non-invasive treatments of alternative medicine — and the patient has an exceptional physician worth his or her weight in gold.

A doctor who genuinely appreciates and practices high quality alternative medicine is a doctor committed to a holistic approach to health care. Their practice is founded on the following "Principles of Ethics" of the American Holistic Medical Association (AHMA):

1. Physicians render service to humanity with full respect for the dignity of humankind, treating the total person: body, mind, and spirit. The treatment shall be at all times in the

best interest of the patient.

2. Physicians continually improve their skill and medical knowledge and make it available to their patients.

3. Physicians recognize that patients have the right to share in making decisions that pertain to their treatment. They guide and educate patients toward this goal and actively encourage patients to share responsibility for their care.

4. A physician has the right to utilize all responsible methods of treatment. The physician has the obligation, however, to determine the efficacy and safety of such procedures and to acquire the skills and training necessary for the delivery of such care. [7]

These principles are at the very core of a healthy alternative/ unconventional medical practice. It is this group of doctors you can trust to practice high quality alternative medicine.

Still, one trend among M.D.'s practicing alternative medicine is *not* good news and that is the tendency of some medical doctors to embrace the *techniques* of alternative medicine without the *spirit* and *ethos* of a holistic approach to health care. This particular group of doctors who call themselves "alternative medical doctors" define alternative medicine simply as any treatment "not widely taught at U.S. medical schools or generally available at U.S. hospitals." [8] Patients who are treated by these physicians have no guarantee that such a doctor using alternative treatments will also treat them in the spirit of a holistic approach to health care. Such a doctor may not treat their patients as human beings or even be interested in their thoughts and feelings about treatment. These doctors, even though they may be using alternative/unconventional techniques, may still see you only as a diagnosis — not as a person.

The fact is that this can be true for *any* practitioner of *any* alternative medical treatments, not just medical doctors. The difference is that most practitioners of alternative medical systems and modalities are, more often than not, committed to the ethos of the holistic approach to health care. They are taught to use this approach as the rationale for the application of the *techniques* of alternative medicine in which they are trained.

In other words, because most systems and modalities of alternative medicine are rooted in an ethos similar to those outlined above by the AHMA, the chances are much higher that a practitioner trained in an alternative system or modality of healing will have incorporated an appreciation for these ethics as part of their training and have a deep commitment to them in his or her practice.

This may not be the case for the Western-trained conventional biomedical doctor who, historically, has had no training in applying the principles that make up the *ethos* of a holistic approach to health care. In fact, some conventional doctors are now taking courses to learn the *techniques* of alternative medicine without training to appreciate the *ethos* of holistic approach to treatment so vital for the healthy application of alternative treatments.

Butch Levy, M.D., L.Ac., of Lakewood, Colorado, and a competently trained and licensed acupuncturist, agrees and says, "Most western doctors have a hard time letting go of their Western paradigm, which is the basis of their medical education, so they can really learn a new way of healing. If they cannot do this, even for a little while, they cannot gain a new understanding. They need to learn to say, 'I understand this concept. Now I have to go on and learn a different way to think as opposed to adapting alternative medicine to how Western medicine thinks it should be.'" [9]

Regrettably, a lot of Western doctors are afraid to do this — to learn another system of medicine on the terms on which it was developed. In order for M.D.'s to practice "high quality" alternative medicine, they have to be willing to change not only what they have been doing, but also how they view the body, what healing is, and the role that a patient plays in the healing process.

Dr. Levy made an initial commitment to do just that when he began studying Chinese medicine. He says, "When I studied Chinese medicine, I made a commitment to myself not to bring a Western paradigm to my study. I went into it saying, 'I don't know anything about this. I have to be willing to start over again. I am going to learn this based on how the Oriental people view this, rather than trying to turn this medicine into conventional medicine or "Western" medicine using Eastern concepts.'" [10]

Unfortunately the broad scope of practice granted to an M.D. by their license allows them to take short, consolidated courses on complex systems of alternative medicine and then immediately offer them to the public. Dr. Levy feels, "No one, not even an M.D., can just take a weekend course in acupuncture and really call him- or herself a competent acupuncturist. I think this practice of M.D.'s taking quick classes and then practicing alternative techniques without responsible training is an important issue for both the public and the state licensing bodies to look at." [11]

Another trend to watch for is the increasing number of alternative medical clinics being run by an M.D. as the oversight physician, with a variety of alternative practitioners such as acupuncturists, chiropractors, massage therapists and body workers, herbalists, and others all working under the authority of the M.D. According to Robert Duggan, M.Ac., Dipl.Ac. (NCCA), who teaches "The Philosophy and Practice of Healing" at Johns Hopkins School of Medicine, this approach is "the wave to come, be it for good or ill." [12] Many worry that if the M.D. is not committed to overseeing an alternative clinic that is founded on the spirit and ethos of a holistic approach to health care, then such a clinic could become a patient mill that fails to provide high quality alternative medical care. Fortunately, there are a growing number of M.D.'s who are committed to the spirit and ethos of holistic approach to health care and many of them will oversee these developing alternative medical clinics. Still, it is in your best interest to do the Five Step process outlined in Part I of this book to be sure you receive high quality alternative medicine when considering treatment at such a clinic.

Here are two stories about two very different alternative medical doctors:

Jessica's Story: Why I Now Believe in Alternative Medical Doctors

Two years ago, I was in bad car accident. I had injuries to my right knee, a broken collar bone, as well as a concussion and "internal bruising." After two surgeries on my knee, I took a month off work to heal my other injuries. But at the end of the month, I did not feel back to my old self.

Five months after the accident, my back and neck were still hurting me; my body was stiff and bruised-feeling; my right knee was still causing me problems; my digestive system did not seem to work right; and, worst of all, I was having a recurring nightmare of the accident and at times had episodes of unexpected terror when riding in or driving a car. No matter what I did, I felt "out of sorts" all the time. My body just did not feel right.

My older brother knew about all this and suggested I see an M.D. he said might be able to help me. He said that this doctor was into "different things" than most medical doctors but assured me that he was not a quack. Given that I had a lot of respect for my brother, I decided to go see this doctor.

When I went to this doctor's office, I was given some papers to read. One was an article on alternative medicine and another was on holistic medicine. I read the information in the articles and many of the ideas were new to me. Still, I especially liked the idea that I would be seen by my doctor as a human being rather than a diagnosis and that the doctor would want to really hear my thoughts and feelings about my health condition.

When the doctor came into the examination room, he greeted me with a warm "Hello!" along with a smile and a handshake.

He sat down and asked me to tell him why I was there to see him. As I told him my story, I was amazed at how he listened to me: he *really* listened. Afterwards, he asked me some questions about my personal life and about my job, as well as how I was doing generally. Next he gave me a physical examination with special attention to the auto injuries. He was very gentle and told me to let him know if anything he was doing was causing me pain. When he finished the physical, he shared with me some of the treatments that he thought would be good for me based on the exam and what I had told him.

He talked about the idea of a "healing program" that would help me really get over the effects of the auto accident. First he discussed what we could do for my body. As part of the healing program, he suggested I take a beginning hatha yoga class to stretch out my tightened muscles and to massage my internal organs. He said that would help me let go of some of the trauma my body was holding onto from the accident as well as possibly help my digestive system to work better. He also told me about homeopathy and said he had some homeopathic remedies that could help the bruised feeling inside my body and even help with my digestion. Next he talked about the terror episodes I was having and told me that this was a normal reaction after such a traumatic event. He suggested another homeopathic remedy for this as well as three to six sessions of Eye Movement Desensitization Reprocessing (EMDR). These sessions would focus on the accident and help me learn to let go of the trauma that was causing the terror episodes.

After sharing his recommendations, this doctor asked me if I had any questions or concerns about his ideas for a healing program. I thought for a minute and told him I was somewhat familiar with yoga, but asked him to explain to me exactly how the homeopathic medicine worked and what EMDR was. The information he shared with me about homeopathy and EMDR was new but seemed to make sense. He gave me several articles and a brochure to help me understand them both even better.

He told me that even though he could not absolutely guarantee it, he believed I could expect to feel at least 75 percent better in about three or four months if I did the whole program. He then asked me if I would be interested in doing the healing program as he had described. I told him I was.

To my surprise, he then asked me if there was anything I could think of that would be good to include in my "healing program." I thought for a moment and said it would probably help if I stopped eating as much junk food and added more "rabbit food" into my diet. He laughed and agreed and offered to give me some information on the power of foods to cause illness or to heal.

After that, he asked me a few more questions, all of which seemed *very* strange to me. Like: Did I crave sweets or fatty foods most? Was I bothered by drafts? What time of day was the hardest for me? How did I feel about being in groups of people? What time of night did my nightmares usually take place? Was there a particular time of day that I got my terror reactions in a car?

I answered his questions and he explained that my answers were helping him to determine exactly which homeopathic remedies would be best for me.

He then got up and went over to the cabinet and took some small white pills out of a bottle and put them in a small envelope for me. He also gave me a small bottle with an eye dropper that also had homeopathic medicine in it. He wrote down the instructions as to how I was to take the medicines. Then he walked me out to the front office where he told his assistant to schedule my EMDR sessions and to give me a list of yoga instructors in town that offered the kind of class he suggested.

The last thing he did was to thank me for coming in. He asked me to remember that we were partners in my healing program and that if it was to work I had to be sure to do my part by taking a beginning yoga class, taking the homeopathic medicines as prescribed, doing the EMDR sessions, and eating more "rabbit food." Also, I was to come back in two weeks to review my progress with him and to feel free to call if I had any questions or concerns. I thanked him and, without even thinking about it, gave him a hug. I was embarrassed by my behavior until he told me that "hugs are spoken freely in this office."

I did the whole healing program for three and a half months and can honestly say I did feel tremendously better. My nightmares have stopped. I do not feel that bruised feeling anymore. And my body is now very supple and relaxed. My knee is also much improved and I have not had a terror episode while riding in a car for four weeks. I have even signed up for an intermediate yoga class and have started to meditate. I still eat some junk food but have really learned to enjoy and appreciate the "rabbit food."

It is obvious that Jessica was fortunate to find a medical doctor not just trained in the techniques of alternative medicine, but also fully committed to practicing the spirit of holistic medicine.

Nathan's Story: The Alternative Doctor I'll Never See Again

I enjoy playing tennis any chance I can. It is not only a way for me to keep fit, but it is also a way for me to enjoy being with my friends. One weekend, as I was moving to return a difficult serve, I felt a sharp pain. I felt it strongly as I tried to move my arm at the elbow joint. It was obvious to me (and everyone else) that I may have done some serious damage and would not be on the courts for awhile.

An acquaintance suggested I go see their doctor, who specialized in sports injuries and also was into "alternative medicine." My friend felt that maybe this doctor's alternative treatments might help my arm heal faster. I did not like the idea of being off the courts for a prolonged period of time, so I decided to give this doctor a try.

I felt fortunate that I was able to get into see him the next day. I arrived at his office and was given the usual paperwork to fill out. After about fifteen minutes, a nurse escorted me into a treatment room and curtly told me to undress and to put on the robe that was hanging on the hook. Though somewhat startled by this instruction, I did as requested.

A few minutes later the doctor came in. Immediately, he walked over and picked up my chart and began to read my intake form. He never looked at me or even said, "Hello." Next, he walked over to me and, without asking or saying anything, took my right arm and moved it toward him so he could look at it. The pain was excruciating. And I let him know it! His only comment was, "Oh, that hurts?" After looking at my elbow and determining that I was *really* in pain, he went over to the counter and got some needles. Without ever saying a word about what he was going to do, he stuck five needles in my right arm at various places. Some of the needles were very painful. Not once did he say anything. Not only that, then he left the room and left me just sitting there with those five damn needles in my arm! About twenty minutes later he came back and took the needles out. While he was making some notes in my chart, he said he wanted to see me in five days to do another treatment. I smiled politely as he then left the room.

After I left his office, I noticed that my arm was not quite as sore as before and I could even move it a little better. But what I noticed most of all was my rage.

I had never been treated by any doctor with such disrespect. I mean, even the doctors in the Marines were more humane than this guy. Even though I did feel some improvement in my arm, there was no way I was going back to see this "alternative" doctor again.

Fortunately, there are not many doctors that would treat a patient with such disrespect. Still, Nathan's story makes an important point: just because a medical doctor is trained in the *techniques* of alternative medicine is no guarantee that that treatment will be done in the *spirit* of a holistic approach to treatment.

The Four Most Popular Ways M.D.'s Package Their Practice of Alternative Medicine

Many of the basic principles and techniques of alternative medicine as practiced by medical doctors are being packaged under a number of different labels for the 1990s. The most popular of these are holistic medicine, alternative medicine, complementary medicine, and integrative medicine. Some other popular labels describing alternative treatments include environmental medicine and preventive medicine. (These labels are not just being used by medical doctors to describe their alternative practices. Many other alternative practitioners, including acupuncturists, naturopaths, chiropractors, and even massage therapists, have taken to describing what they do as holistic, alternative, complementary, or integrative health care.)

No matter how an M.D. labels his or her practice, it is still critical that you make sure that they are competently trained in the nonconventional treatments they practice and that they are committed to practicing in the spirit and ethos of a holistic approach. By doing this, you can be assured of getting high quality alternative medical care.

Holistic medicine, alternative medicine, conventional medicine, and integrative medicine all advocate the use of alternative/unconventional medical treatments, but where they differ is in the role such treatments play in relationship to conventional medicine.

Holistic Medicine

Holistic physicians are conventionally trained doctors who have chosen to go beyond the basic biomedical philosophical underpinnings of their training as "doctors." They have opened their hearts and minds to include an appreciation of other medicines from different cultures, different times, and different philosophies in their commitment to "treat the whole person."

The American Holistic Medical Association (AHMA) defines holistic medicine: "This emerging medical specialty is an art and science that treats and prevents disease, while focusing on empowering patients to create a condition of optimal health. Far more than the absence of illness, this state of health is a dynamic balance of the physical, environmental, mental, emotional, social, and spiritual aspects of an individual. As both a healer and health educator, the holistic physician, in partnership with the patient, addresses the causes of disease in addition to treating its symptoms."[13]

Interestingly, the initial integration of the *spirit and ethos* of the holistic approach to health care as an influential force in modern conventional biomedical practices began in the late 1950s and early 1960s with the advent of the holistic medical movement. Though its influence was slow in creating real changes in health care, the changes are steadily increasing and continue to this day.

Many feel that this process formally began with the personal search of one man, Evarts Loomis, M.D., F.A.C.S.I., often called "the father of holistic medicine." In 1940, while on assignment in Newfoundland, Dr. Loomis had a dream. "One night I awoke with the words, 'Treat the whole person,' echoing through my mind," he says. "I saw that there were spiritual, emotional, as well as physical, aspects of man and that they all needed to be looked at during illness. I saw that I had just been treating the effects of illness. Right then I decided to investigate all aspects of man to find the causes of illness."[14]

This concept was unheard of in the conventional medicine of the 1940s and 1950s and so, on their own, Dr. Loomis and his wife Vera nurtured this dream. In 1958 they founded "Meadowlark," considered the first holistic medical retreat center in the United States.

Dr. Loomis developed a basic program that included a thorough physical examination and such treatments as nutritional counseling, exercise, homeopathic medicine, acupuncture, therapeutic fasts, hatha yoga, art and music therapy, and psycho-spiritual counseling, with daily group therapy sessions incorporating the use of dreams, Progoffian journaling, and instruction in meditative techniques.

Dr. Loomis observed that during an illness the emotions and the mind played an important role in the healing process. So guests at Meadowlark worked to heal resentments through forgiveness techniques and journaled on the meaning of their lives, and considered why their illness had come to them and what it had to teach them. The word patient wasn't used, and staff were not distinguished from the guests by white coats.

"Through fifty some years of practice, and more than 6,000 Meadowlark guests, I have seen many dramatic healings that defy orthodox Western medicine," Dr. Loomis says. "I came to understand that there were no incurable diseases, just incurable minds." [15]

Patients to this day still seek out Dr. Loomis for his assistance. Just recently, a woman from Chicago called Dr. Loomis. She had been to Meadowlark six times while it was under his direction. She had originally come to Meadowlark to heal a terminal lung cancer condition. Through Dr. Loomis's program, it went into remission. Now, twelve years later, her cancer returned but had not spread. She called to say how grateful she was for those twelve years of remission and asked, "Could Dr. Loomis help again?" At eighty-six, Dr. Loomis is still active as a lecturer, teacher, and counselor with his partner, Fay L. Loomis.

By the 1970s, Dr. Loomis's principles of holistic medicine were beginning to be appreciated and then practiced by a small but dedicated group of medical doctors. In 1978, Norman Shealy, M.D., and some of these doctors founded the American Holistic Medical Association (AHMA). Today, there are a respectable number of medical doctors who describe their practice of alternative/unconventional treatments as holistic medicine.

Alternative Medicine

In the mid-1980s the term "alternative medicine" began to gain popularity. Today, it is now more recognized and used by the public and the press when referring to nonconventional medical health care treatments than the terms holistic, complementary, or integral.

Usually, medical doctors who describe themselves as alternative medical doctors see their practices as an "alternative" to regular conventional medicine. To many of these doctors, alternative implies an either/or situation in treatment: that either unconventional treatments are used *or* conventional medicine is used.

For medical doctors who use the label of "alternative medicine" to describe their medical practices, alternative can mean two very different things: (1) That they are essentially the same as the holistic doctor in their philosophy of treatment and are committed to practicing in the spirit and ethos of a holistic approach to health care in the application of alternative treatments (high quality alternative medicine) or, (2) that they use treatments that are an "alternative" to conventional medicine — not generally taught at U.S. medical schools — while *not* incorporating the spirit and ethos of a holistic approach to health care.

Given this, it is important to verify a doctor's competency in alternative treatments and also to make sure they are committed to including the spirit and ethos of a holistic approach in their practice.

Complementary Medicine

Beginning in the 1990s, a growing number of doctors and hospitals began to describe their use of unconventional and alternative medical treatments as complementary medicine. The emphasis was on using nonconventional treatments as a *complement* to already prescribed conventional medical treatment.

Different from the "either/or" nuance of the "alternative" label for medical treatment, in complementary medicine, nonconventional treatments are used as an *adjunct* to conventional treatments. The conventional medical treatments are the primary form of treatment while other systems of medicine, modalities, and nonconventional treatments play a *secondary role* to support and complement the conventional medical treatment.

Author Larry Dossey, M.D., shares a personal experience with a patient who requested her own form of complementary medicine when he was in practice as an internist several years ago. "I had a patient who had an enlarged ovary and needed surgery because we were concerned it might be cancerous," he says. "This woman had a very sophisticated, complex view of the world that I really admired and shared. As I was sorting through all the gynecologists who I could refer her to, the question in my mind was, 'Who in the world am I going to ask to operate on this woman?' My patient strongly believed in the power of music, of hypnosis, of pyramids, and that only positive things be said to her while she was under anesthesia.

"I thought of one woman gynecologist who I thought would be open to working within the belief systems of this woman. So I asked the physician, 'Can you honor this patient's beliefs about healing even though they may be very different than your own?' The doctor felt that she could. Then I asked the same question of the anesthesiologist and the nursing staff. Everyone said that they would cooperate.

"When my patient arrived at her room at the hospital, she set up a sound system and played music she felt would help her heal. She made other changes to the room, including hanging art work from her home so she could have the kind of visual input in a sterile room that she felt was important to her.

"She had the surgery as scheduled and it went very well. The most impressive result was that she was released about three days ahead of prediction. Also worthy of note: The gynecologist and the entire staff learned a tremendous amount about how these things can really help a patient." [16]

The term "complementary care" is now being used to describe the philosophy of treatment of a number of progressive and innovative hospitals and clinics. Special emphasis has been placed on utilizing this approach with cancer patients at such institutions as Columbia-Presbyterian Medical Center,

Memorial Sloan-Kettering Cancer Center, Commonweal Cancer Help Program, and Duke Comprehensive Cancer Center.[17] In some programs, Ayurveda, behavioral medicine, Chinese medicine, chiropractic, energy medicine, environmental medicine, homeopathy, Native American medicine, naturopathic medicine, nutritional medicine, and osteopathic medicine are being used as adjuncts to conventional medical treatments.[18] Some of the more popular "complementary treatments" include meditation and other stress reduction techniques, i.e., biofeedback, therapeutic massage/therapeutic touch, herbal medicine, and prayer therapy.

Integrative Medicine

The most recent of the more popular terms being used to describe the use of unconventional/alternative treatments by medical doctors and other health care practitioners, is integrative medicine (sometimes also called "integral medicine"). Andrew Weil, M.D., director of the Program in Integrative Medicine at the University of Arizona Medical School and author of *Spontaneous Healing* (Knopf, 1995), has suggested that our current system of medical education be overhauled so that our future doctors can learn alternative systems of medicine and healing with a full appreciation of the healing power of nature and other holistic principles as part of their training.

Integrative medicine seeks to recognize and appreciate the value and wisdom of all healing and medical traditions, giving each their due respect. Different than complementary medicine, which emphasizes the use of unconventional treatments as an adjunct to conventional medicine, integrative medicine seeks to utilize whatever modalities and treatments are the most effective, without preference to any one system, for treating the health care needs of the patients.

Dr. Butch Levy, medical doctor and licensed acupuncturist, says, "A lot of people take herbs and also take their Western medicines. I think that is fine. Crossover is not a problem. It's not about which system of medicine is better than the other. It is about what works." [19]

Medical doctors who practice integrative medicine advocate a combination approach to treatment, including mainstream medicine and nonconventional treatments such as homeopathy, acupuncture, *and* herbal medicine. No favorable bias is given to any one system of medicine, modality, or treatment. All are looked at without prejudice with only one question in mind, "Which systems, modalities, or treatments are the best to use for the patient's condition?"

Leonard Wisneski, M.D., medical director for the Marriott Corporation, says, "Integral medicine combines the best of conventional, alternative, and wellness medicines and is the structure for the future of health care." [21] There is a growing interest in this approach by the public and also the medical community. Dr. Levy agrees. "I think there are a lot of physicians who have really opened their minds a little more to trying to embrace other philosophies of medicine," he says. "It's what the public wants. People want something other than just conventional medicine." [20]

Given the rapidly growing appreciation for other systems of medicine and the increasing body of research that verifies their efficacy, it is quite likely that "integrative medicine" is truly the medicine of the future.

HEALTH CONDITIONS THAT RESPOND BEST TO AN M.D. USING ALTERNATIVE MEDICINE

Increasingly the public and conventional doctors recognize that conventional medicine alone does not have all the answers to our health care needs. There is also a growing appreciation for the role that unconventional/alternative treatments can play to address this problem. This is especially so when it comes to chronic health conditions and end-stage illnesses.

Dr. Levy says, "I have found that most physicians that deal with chronic problems that they can't solve usually are more open to me as an alternative medical doctor than physicians who deal with acute-care medicine. I think that physicians who have been in practice a while, treating chronic illness, debilitating diseases, and end-stage illnesses (cancer, kidney disease, liver disease) realize that what they have to offer really does not get these people well." [22]

As mentioned earlier, the use of alternative treatments for cancer is now being incorporated as an adjunct to conventional medicine in many respected hospitals and clinics as "complementary medicine" or "complementary care." "I have a lot of specialists who are willing to send me their patients because they are frustrated and they don't know what to do," Dr. Levy says. "For example I had one oncologist say to me, 'You know I have been in practice twenty-five years doing this and it is really apparent that what I do is not very satisfactory to a lot of people. If you have a better way of approaching it, I am certainly willing to listen to that approach because I realize what I do doesn't offer everything.' I think this is good example of what is starting to change in medicine." [23]

Applying the Five Steps to the M.D. as an Alternative Practitioner

Additions to Step Two: Get Good Referrals

The oldest association representing physicians who practice alternative medicine is the American Holistic Medical Association (AHMA). Their members and officers represent some of the most visible and respected medical providers of alternative medicine in this country, including: Bernie Siegel, M.D.; Jonathan Collin, M.D., editor of the *Townsend Letter*; Christiane Northrup, M.D.; Deepak Chopra, M.D.; and Andrew Weil, M.D.

If you are looking for a competent alternative medical doctor, the American Holistic Medical Association will provide you with some good prospects to investigate. The AHMA will give you the names of practicing doctors in your area who are members of their association. Although they are good candidates, the referrals are not offered with a guarantee. Also the American Holistic Health Association (AHHA) in Anaheim, California, has a comprehensive referral network.

Another source of good referrals is the American College of Advancement in Medicine in Laguna Hills, California. It provides information and a referral list of M.D.'s around the world trained in preventive medicine, including chelation therapy.

Consider checking with American Academy of Environmental Medicine (AAEM), which has a network of over six hundred physicians practicing a variety of alternative medical treatments. To find M.D.'s trained in homeopathy, contact the National Center for Homeopathy and ask for their referral list. You can also find referrals through the American Preventive Medical Association, an advocacy organization with physicians, other alternative practitioners, and the public as members. The Price-Pottinger Foundation in San Diego, California, is also an excellent referral source.

Additions to Step Three: Screen the Candidates

Once you have found an alternative medical doctor who interests you, call his or her office. You can gather a tremendous amount of valuable information by asking the right questions of the doctor's office staff. Here are some suggestions:

Will you describe the doctor's training in any techniques he or she didn't learn in medical school?

Be sure to find out the number of hours of training the doctor has had in each technique. In addition, ask for board or organizational certifications of completion and competency.

For example, medical doctors who have incorporated acupuncture into their conventional practice might experience success in treating certain conditions that their conventional training alone would not afford them, such as acute and chronic pain that had not responded to conventional medical treatments.

Be careful of the doctors practicing acupuncture with only a small amount of training. A board-certified acupuncturist is required to have over fifteen hundred hours of training. The difference between the experience of being treated by a week-end-seminar acupuncturist and a well-trained, certified acupuncturist can be dramatic.

Regarding M.D.'s who practice homeopathy, Maesimund Panos, M.D., a homeopathic physician and coauthor of *Homeopathic Medicine at Home* (Jeremy P. Tarcher, 1981), says, "The answer you don't want to hear is that they were trained in self-help study groups. Study groups are great, but you want your homeopathic care to come from a professional." [24]

To determine how much training an M.D. should have to competently treat you with a specific alternative technique, call the technique's professional association [see Reference Section] and ask for their standards of competence. Associations and trade organizations representing osteopathic manipulation or Chinese medical techniques, for example, expect M.D.'s to earn hundreds of hours of training from educational facilities specializing in their technique in order to meet minimum competence levels.

How long has the doctor been using these alternative treatments?

Better to be treated by someone who has had the time and hours to mature in the practice and use of his or her chosen alternative treatments than to have a physician "practicing" on you. If the physician has very few hours of training in alternative treatments and is just beginning to use them on his or her patients, you might want to find another physician.

What success has the doctor had in treating patients with physical problems similar to mine?

If you have a specific condition to correct, knowing the doctor's track record will be a significant factor in deciding to work with this physician or not. Ask to have a few patients call you who have had similar problems which the doctor has successfully helped. Generally, if patients are happy with their results, they are apt to share them.

Additions to Step Four: Interview the Provider

Do you practice a holistic approach to health care? If so, what does that exactly mean to you?

If this physician has no interest in practicing in the spirit of holistic health care, you'll know immediately from his or her answer to this question. If the physician does practice holistically, he or she will be happy to share with you exactly what that means to them. Such information can help you decide if they are the right doctor for you.

Do you practice alternative techniques exclusively or in tandem with conventional medicine?

The answer to this question should give you an indication of how much alternative medicine the physician uses in his or her practice and if they are alternative, complementary, or integral in their approach.

Can you describe your training in the alternative techniques you use and how long you have used them?

If you feel you did not get a complete answer to this question from the staff, ask it again of the physician. It is critical that you are confident that this physician is competent in the alternative practices he or she uses before agreeing to treatment.

Additions to Step Five: Form a Partnership

First and foremost, recognize that even though the person sitting across from you is the "doctor," he or she is also a human being like you. To get the most out of your relationship with this professional, you would be wise to respect this person and to recognize their feelings and concerns about your situation.

Also, it is important to understand that this physician has been trained for years to believe that he or she is the responsible party. Even if your doctor is clearly committed to the spirit of a holistic approach to treatment, he or she has professional and licensing constraints to which he or she still must be sensitive. Dr. Christiane Northrup explains, "It's difficult in a medical situation where you are the doctor. You're expected to know everything and not make a mistake. No matter what happens, it's your fault. So it's going to be difficult to give the reins or part of the reins over to your patients." [26]

Still, it is important that you communicate exactly what you need and want, as well as what you do not want, so you can determine if this is the doctor for you. When working with a physician, Bernie Siegel, M.D., says, "I am inflexible about how I'm treated. I want to be treated like a human being — with respect. Also, I want to work with someone who is vulnerable enough to say, 'I'm sorry,' when things go wrong." [25]

WHAT TO EXPECT DURING AN APPOINTMENT WITH AN M.D. AS AN ALTERNATIVE MEDICINE PROVIDER

Most M.D.'s begin their initial appointment with a patient by taking a basic medical history and completing a routine physical exam. From this point, your appointment with an M.D. who practices alternative medicine can go in a variety of different directions, depending on what alternative treatments are provided and whether he or she is alternative, holistic, complementary, or integrative in how he or she uses alternative treatments.

If the M.D. has training in homeopathy, then a more extensive period of questioning, about everything from your sleeping habits to your favorite foods, will generally occur before a remedy is prescribed. If the M.D. uses manipulative therapies, he or she might lightly touch your back to find areas of swelling or tenderness.

Whatever modality of alternative medicine a physician uses, do some research before your first appointment so you are familiar with the treatments the physician may use. This research can be especially valuable to you if the physician gives you a choice of which therapies you'd like him or her to do. Dr. Levy says, "With my patients, I explain that there are different models of medicine and healing, and different ways of treating. Then I present them with a choice. I say, 'This is what I can do. Here are the things that you can choose from.' I will say, 'This is an allopathic [biomedical] approach and here is what it will do and not do for you. If you are interested in an alternative, here are some other treatments that I do and here is what they will do and not do for you.' "[27]

You may find in your experience with alternative medicine that the results do not take place as fast as the results from conventional medicine. Patients who are suffering from chronic illnesses need an extra dosage of patience regarding alternative medicine because they may not see marked change for six months or more. However, the advantage is that, in such cases, alternative medicine will probably have addressed the cause and made definite headway in permanently healing the condition.

Some doctors who take a more integrative approach to alternative medical treatment may initially address the symptoms and after address the deeper causes. "Usually I have to treat people initially for the problem, the symptoms, because in order to be credible I have to produce some relief," Dr. Levy says. "And the truth is they are entitled to this relief. Over time, this builds trust and confidence and then I can say to them, 'We treated the problem — the symptoms — now we have go deeper and treat the pattern that created the problem — the cause — or else the problem will just return.' "[28]

An appointment with an M.D. who practices alternative medicine can include conversations ranging from the benefits of surgery to the value to be gained from "laying on of hands" or prayer therapy. There is a very wide range of treatments you may be offered. Given this, your best tactic is to gather as much information about the physician, especially their qualifications, to give you those treatments.

COST AND INSURANCE

Cost

A visit to an M.D. practicing alternative medicine may or may not be similar to what you would pay a regular medical doctor. Sometimes it will actually cost you less, because the treatments do not require medical tests and are fairly simple procedures. Other times the cost can be much higher because extensive testing may be required and/or the treatments, by their nature, are costly. Given this, you would be wise to ask *before* treatment what procedures are usually involved for your condition and what they usually cost.

Insurance

Although all M.D.'s and most of their conventional treatments are covered by insurance plans if they are found to be medically necessary, not all plans cover M.D.'s performing alternative medical treatments. Even though more and more plans are covering some alternative treatments, such as acupuncture, biofeedback, and homeopathy, most plans still do not. For this reason, it is important to check with your insurance carrier to see if they will pay for your alternative medical treatments and, if so, under what circumstances.

However, research indicates that many people are still willing to try alternative treatments even if they aren't covered by their health insurance plans. "The biggest issue is cost," Dr. Levy says. "If their insurance doesn't cover alternative treatments, it is difficult for people sometimes to afford it. Still, even with this the majority of my patients are open to trying it." [29]

EDUCATION, TRAINING, AND LICENSING

The titles or labels of alternative M.D., holistic M.D., complementary M.D., or integral M.D. are self-proclaimed and purely voluntary. No special courses are required and no tests are administered to demonstrate competency. It is in your best interest to determine what you can expect from your doctor *before* your first appointment.

All M.D.'s are educated and trained in conventional biomedical philosophy and procedures in medical school. Training for competency in alternative treatments is not yet a part of that process — nor is training in the spirit of the holistic approach to health care, as discussed throughout this chapter. Dr. Norman

Shealy, founding president of the American H[
Association, says, "Training [in alternative hea
niques] is the greatest weakness of the whole h⌣...
tive] movement because there are no residencies. There aren't
even any fellowships of any significance. So virtually all of
the holistic [alternative] physicians have trained themselves
through special post-graduate work." [30] How much training the
doctor believes he or she should have in order to be competent
is a decision each one makes for him- or herself. Whether the
doctor's standards for competency in a particular alternative
treatment are as high as yours is a decision for you to make.

Fortunately, the American Holistic Medical Association
(AHMA) is sensitive to this issue and has recently established
the American Board of Holistic Medicine (ABHM) ... "for the purpose of certifying physicians as practitioners of holistic medicine." [31] The exam an applicant must take to become certified
consists of seven core knowledge areas: nutrition, physical activity, environmental medicine, behavioral medicine, social health,
energy medicine, and spiritual attunement. It will also cover six
secondary subjects: botanical medicine, homeopathy, ethno-
medicine (traditional Chinese medicine, Ayurveda, Native American medicine), manual medicine (manipulation, body work,
etc.), biomolecular therapies, and health promotion. Further, "In
addition to the board examination, the certification process will
include an interview, a self-administered test of holistic health,
and a minimum of six years in active medical practice (which can
include residency training)." [32] Such trends in conventional medicine are welcome, given the public interest and desire for high
quality alternative medical care.

In many states, conventional medical doctors, just by the
broad scope of their license to practice, can provide alternative
treatments that they have not been required to demonstrate
competency in. There are exceptions to this. For example, in New
Mexico, licensed medical doctors must have a separate license
to practice acupuncture. This means that all M.D.'s practicing
Chinese medicine in New Mexico have to pass the same exam

that is required of graduates of four-year Chinese medical schools, who have had over fifteen hundred hours of study to their credit. Some other states place minimum requirements of hours studied, ranging from two hundred to one thousand hours.

In Arizona, in order for M.D.'s or D.O.'s to legally practice homeopathy, they must take a separate exam from their regular license to demonstrate competency in homeopathic medicine.

Many feel that these kinds of requirements of medical doctors will be a growing trend in other states to protect people seeking competent high quality alternative medical treatment from medical doctors.

CLOSING THOUGHTS

M.D.'s who are well trained in conventional medicine, embrace a holistic approach to health care, and have competent training in alternative medical treatments, are unquestionably some of the finest health care providers in the profession.

It is these doctors that deserve special recognition because they have also been, and still are, courageous pioneers who have faced the scrutiny and criticism of their peers to speak out about the value of alternative medical systems so different from their original, conventional medical training.

It is still true today that the health care professional whose opinion is most respected and listened to is the M.D. For that reason, M.D.'s who have placed their businesses and professional reputations at risk to speak about the importance of the spirit of a holistic approach to health care and the value of alternative therapies are nothing short of heroes and heroines.

Chapter 7

TRADITIONAL CHINESE MEDICINE

Harmonizing the Opposites, Unleashing the Power

Human life is the gathering of chi ... if it disperses, one is no more.

– Chuang Zi, Taoist sage

DID YOU KNOW THAT:

- One quarter of the world's population uses one or more Chinese medical therapies. [1]

- An estimated twelve million patients in the United States visit practitioners of Chinese medicine every year. [2]

- There are more than fifty schools in the U.S. training practitioners of Chinese medicine. [3]

- There are over seven thousand practitioners of Chinese medicine practicing in the U.S. today. [4]

- Twenty-two states license, register, or certify practitioners of Chinese medicine for independent practice. [5]

- The National Institutes of Health's Office of Alternative Medicine has funded ten research studies on Chinese medical treatments from 1993 to 1994. [6]

- The U.S. Government has spent over $1 million in research funding to study Chinese medicine's success in treating substance abuse. [7]

- More than twenty hospitals in the U.S. use acupuncture in

their addiction treatment programs. [8]

• Controlled research studies have shown compelling evidence of acupuncture's efficacy in osteoarthritis, chemotherapy-induced nausea, asthma, back pain, painful menstrual cycles, bladder instability, and migraine headaches. [9]

• Former Surgeon General C. Everett Koop, M.D., has recognized acupuncture as a useful method of overcoming nicotine addiction. [10]

The Basic Principles of Chinese Medicine

Based on Oriental philosophy, the Chinese medical concepts defining how the human body operates, becomes ill, and heals are foreign to most Westerners. Whereas Western medicine is linear, scientific, and founded in Cartesian-Newtonian science, Chinese medicine draws its strength from intuition and observation and takes its precepts from the natural world. Chinese medicine is rooted in the idea that "the human being is a microcosm, a universe in miniature, the offspring of Heaven and Earth, a fusion of cosmic and terrestrial forces." [11] Chinese medicine is based on subtle, yet complex, principles, all sourced from observations of nature. "A postulate of Chinese medicine is that by observing patterns in the natural world, the dynamics of human nature are known. As above, so below." [12] Chinese medicine speaks in a language of metaphors that comes from conditions found in nature. These metaphors become evident in typical diagnoses of Chinese medicine. For example a diagnosis might read, "Deficient fire to the kidneys and dampness in the lungs." Health is evaluated through the prisms of two primary oriental concepts, "chi" (vital energy) and "yin-yang." Chi is described by the National Accreditation Commission for Schools and Colleges of Acupuncture and Oriental Medicine (NACSCAOM) in Washington, D.C., as "energy present and flowing within the universe and within each person. Chi energy circulates through the body in well-defined cycles, moving in a prescribed sequence from point to point. Traditional acupuncture has mapped twelve primary (and eight secondary) pathways or meridians along which the chi energy travels.... The healing techniques of acupuncture and Oriental medicine affect the flow and intensity of chi energy. Like a tightrope walker, the chi energy must remain balanced as it moves forward." [13] It is the intent of the Chinese medical practitioner to move chi forward harmoniously.

The dynamic of yin/yang is the harmony of the opposites. Yin and yang exist as polarities but are not thought of in terms of "either-or" or "negative-positive." In Chinese thought, every condition contains the seeds for its reversal. In fact, the Chinese ideogram (word) for our word "crisis" is actually composed of two symbols: "danger" and "opportunity." Likewise, every underlying physical imbalance is viewed as an opportunity for healing. This approach to polarity as paradox has a connection to healing. Symptoms lead the practitioner of Chinese medicine to an understanding of how the yin and yang elements are out of balance, to the underlying causes of illness and how to unblock the trapped chi. Once released, it becomes a powerful source for recovery and renewal.

The Ancient Roots of Chinese Medicine

Traditional Chinese medicine, also called Oriental medicine, has its origins in ancient China over four thousand years ago. During the Han Dynasty in the second century B.C., it became codified as a comprehensive system of health care. Over the last thousand years, Chinese medicine has spread to all parts of the globe, including Africa, Asia, Europe, India, as well as North, Central, and South America. Also, there is evidence that in the mid-1800s, it was practiced here in the U.S. in Oregon and Idaho by traditional Chinese doctors. [14]

Chinese medicine caught the attention of the modern American public in the 1970s when the United States normalized relations with China. At that time, *New York Times* journalist James Reston required an emergency appendectomy while on assignment in China and made headline news across the country. According to *Time* magazine, "Reston reported that an acupuncturist's needles effectively blocked his pain following the operation." Reston said, "I have seen the past and it works!" For most Americans, the report of Reston's experience was the first time they had ever heard of acupuncture.[15]

Chinese medicine's treatments have successfully helped hundreds of millions of people over its thousands of years of practice. And it still has its applications today, as in Reston's case. In fact, the World Health Organization now recommends Chinese medicine for over one hundred of our modern-day illnesses.[16]

The Major Chinese Medical Treatments

The traditional Chinese doctor uses acupuncture, acupressure, cupping, moxibustion, herbs, food, massage, and exercise to recover and preserve health. These eight major treatments are used either exclusively or in tandem during a session with the Chinese medical practitioner.[17] For example, during a session with her Chinese medical doctor, Mary was given an acupuncture treatment on two areas of her body. Then, because she was battling a respiratory infection, the practitioner also performed cupping on some points on her back. Before she left the office, she was given a bag of Chinese herbs to boil into a tea at home. Also she was told to abstain from foods that were classified in Chinese medicine as "hot." Oily and spicy foods as well as certain fruits like tangerines were part of that list.

Most visits to a traditional Chinese medicine practitioner will include a combination of medical treatments. Below is a more detailed description of the major treatments of Chinese medicine and how they might be used by a Chinese medical practitioner.

Acupuncture is the most widely recognized and the most popular treatment of Chinese medicine. In fact, because of its popularity, some schools of Chinese medicine teach only acupuncture, excluding all other components of Chinese medicine.

Though still held suspect by some Westerners, acupuncture

has not only withstood the test of time, but also the test of the U.S. court system. The following is part of a court decision made by Judge Gabrielle K. McDonald, U.S. District Court for the Southern District of Texas: "Acupuncture has been practiced for two thousand to five thousand years. It is no more experimental as a mode of medical treatment than is the Chinese language as a mode of communication. What is experimental is not acupuncture, but Westerner's understanding of it and their ability to utilize it properly." [18]

Acupuncture stimulates energetic points on the body with the insertion of a slim, sterile acupuncture needle. Acupuncture theory suggests that this stimulation has the potential to create positive change in any aspect of a person's physical, emotional, mental, or spiritual being. In 1979, the World Health Organization listed 104 physical illnesses that acupuncture treatments help to heal, including migraines; sinusitis; asthma; disorders of the eyes, ears, and throat; brain damage; and sciatica. [19]

Acupuncture is currently being used to help heroin or cocaine addicts overcome their addictions. Some jails and prisons have even found that acupuncture on inmates has helped them overcome their tendency to commit criminal acts. According to the *National Acupuncture Detoxification Association Newsletter*, "Women incarcerated in the Santa Barbara, California, county jail who received thirty-two or more acupuncture treatments while in custody had an overall reincarceration rate 26 percent lower than the control group that received no acupuncture. Those who received less than thirty-two treatments had a 17 percent lower rate of incarceration during the first four months after release from jail." [20] Based on these kinds of results, an increasing number of public agencies and criminal justice systems across the United States are taking a genuine interest in acupuncture.

One of the most well-researched applications for acupuncture in the U.S. is for chronic and acute pain. Scores of people have found acupuncture to help relieve debilitating pain, including Francesco Scavullo, a top fashion photographer. He says about his battle with crippling arthritis, "Before [acupuncture from] Dr. Chu, I was living on cortisone, Motrin, Advil and other pills.... Instead of ending up in a wheelchair, I'm skiing and jumping horses."[21]

Acupressure is sometimes considered acupuncture without needles. During acupressure, the same energetic points and channels used in acupuncture are stimulated with touch to produce symptomatic relief. Although it is primarily used for stimulating a healing response in nonemergency circumstances, it can also be effective in crisis situations. Here's a dramatic example from a physician who helped save a man's life through acupressure:

"A patient was brought to our intensive care unit from another hospital emergency room, where he had been given a hundred milligrams of Thorazine (an antipsychotic drug) intramuscularly. Thorazine has a faster and greater effect when injected than when taken orally, but it also has a greater chance of lowering the blood pressure. This man had been given a very high dosage — and the hospital staff hadn't noticed that he was drunk. You *never* mix alcohol and a major antipsychotic because they are addictive in effect.

"When the patient arrived, the medication was just taking effect. He went under before the eyes of the admitting personnel, becoming less responsive and more groggy, then turning gray. When I arrived, his pulse was so weak that I couldn't feel it and the blood pressure was 40/0, which indicates a coronary arrest with imminent danger of dying. By the time we got him into the room, he was totally unresponsive and just whitish gray, like a person looks just before dying due to lack of oxygen.

"I put my knuckle into his sternum and dug in hard to elicit a pain reflex and stimulate adrenaline release, which sometimes can revive a person. Nothing. I didn't have the necessary medical equipment to do some of the things that Western medicine can do because this was a psychiatric unit. Here I was, looking at a guy who was going to have a cardiac arrest at any moment. I could stand by and watch him die or I could do something — anything. I suddenly remembered ... a primary [acupressure] revival point and the most important one for loss of consciousness. So I pulled the patient's shoes off and, without explaining to the nurses what I was doing, proceeded to put my thumbs almost through his feet at these points.

It took about two minutes, three at the most. He started moving around a bit at first and then moaning a little. By the end of those few minutes, he had sat up in his chair and was talking to us. He had a strong pulse and a blood pressure of 90/40. There was an amazed look on the nurses' faces as they asked what I had done. I said I had worked with the acupressure points to mobilize reserved energy. I don't know if that made any sense to them, but they were amazed and happy that the patient was alive. Meanwhile, by the way, a priority code ambulance — with sirens and lights and the whole bit — was on its way to pick up a supposedly dying patient." [22]

As treatments such as acupressure are added to their practices, practitioners and their patients are being pleasantly surprised by the results to their health.

Cupping uses the strength of a vacuum to disperse blocked or congested chi in specific body areas. It is done by warming either a glass or bamboo cup and applying it to particular zones or areas of the body.

A friend of ours shared her story about cupping. She was three months pregnant and fighting a serious case of bronchitis that was threatening to turn into pneumonia. She went to see her Chinese medical practitioner, Ming, because she knew from past experience that this practitioner could handle serious infections without the drugs that would negatively affect her baby. During her appointment with Ming, in addition to acupuncture, three warmed cups were placed on her back. Our friend remembers, "The cupping created such a soothing sensation of warmth and relaxation in places that had felt constricted and tight before the treatment. After Ming gently removed the cups, I noticed immediately that my breathing was noticeably better. After two more of these treatments within a two-week period, my bronchitis was gone."

Because of its effectiveness in reestablishing balance to the meridians by the application of a drawing warmth, cupping is helpful for other conditions, including arthritis and muscle injuries.

Herbal Medicine is a primary modality of Chinese medicine and, in some styles of Chinese medicine, is the only treatment used. Chinese herbs are primarily made of plant material and prescribed to patients to help change a physical condition. Some herbs are chosen to bring specific qualities into the body and to harmonize energy patterns that may be the source of the illness. Other herbs bring nutrition and strength to particular organ systems. The combination of the client's energy and the prescribed herbs brings about synergistic change that supports healing.

Harriet Beinfeld, L.Ac., and Effrem Korngold, L.Ac., authors of *Heaven and Earth: A Guide to Chinese Medicine*, say, "Herbs tend to have greater concentrations of nonnutritive compounds than do foods (i.e., glycosides, resins, alkaloids, polysaccarides, and terpenes), which contribute to their effectiveness as medicine, that is a substance capable of promoting a desirable biologic process or altering a pathologic one." [23] It is theorized that it is these compounds that cause herbs to be so effective in promoting healing.

Moxibustion is older than the use of needles and was at one time considered the preferred treatment. It is a healing technique where a practitioner burns the herb Artemisia vulgaris (a plant of the daisy family, often called "Moxa") on an acupuncture point. According to *Alternative Healing: The Complete A to Z Guide to Over 160 Different Alternative Therapies*, "When ignited, moxa smolders without producing a flame." [24]

The burning herb is intended to warm and stimulate specific energetic points so that a change in the flow of chi occurs to support the necessary healing. When Mary had a session with her acupuncturist, she was surprised to see her practitioner twist moxa on several of her acupuncture needles and light them. She asked the practitioner why she was doing this. Her practitioner replied that Mary's kidney chi was weak after giving birth, and she needed extra stimulation at these points to help her kidney chi return to optimal vitality. Mary thought the burning of this herb would make the needles uncomfortable, but actually the warmth was rather soothing. The treatment was effective, also. As a result of the treatment, her energy level improved significantly.

Nutrition and Diet — Nutrition and dietetic recommendations can also be a part of Chinese medical treatment depending on the illness/imbalance and its seriousness. Foods are suggested based on their energetic properties such as toxifying, dispersing, heating, cooling, moistening, and drying. If, for instance, a client has a fever from an infection, a practitioner of Chinese medicine would recommend cooling foods like watermelon, celery, and cucumber and would also suggest avoiding oily or spicy foods.

Also, practitioners emphasize the value of eating in tune with seasonal changes and life activities. For example, Chinese medical practitioners suggest eating more warming foods such as meats, garlic, and spices during the colder seasons of autumn and winter. A higher ratio of cooler foods such as cold vegetables and raw fruits are recommended during the warmer months of spring and summer. Chinese practitioners also recommend detoxifying diets for short periods of time before the cold of autumn and winter.

Remedial Massage — In traditional Chinese medicine, remedial massage is an ancient touching technique passed down through the generations, which uses two distinctive forms of hand motions, "An-mo" and "Tuina." The "Chantilly Report" to the NIH says, "The techniques of remedial massage (an-mo and tuina) are described in the medical texts of the Han Period. Later in the Tang dynasty, massage was taught in special institutes." [25]

"Tuina" is considered a treatment and strengthens a client's body with rubbing and pressing hand motions. In addition to bringing additional blood flow, this technique also helps to release blocked chi, helping the body to heal and release toxins. The other technique, "An-mo," creates a calming effect with the use of rolling and thrusting motions for relaxation and the relief of tension and stress.

The stimulation created by these manual techniques enhance overall well-being while supporting healing. Conditions such as sprains, headaches, hypertension, and back pain have all been successfully treated with remedial massage.

Qigong is both a physical fitness exercise and a tool for self-healing. Its intention is to enhance, cleanse, and focus the flow of chi through the body to promote health and vitality. This is done by performing a "practice" once a day for twenty to forty minutes.

During a practice, one calms the mind through meditation while consistently regulating one's breathing by performing each choreographed movement with focused attention and by visualizing chi (energy) surging steadily, smoothly, and powerfully through one's body. According to *The American Holistic Health Association Complete Guide to Alternative Medicine,* "It is estimated that 1.3 million residents of Beijing use the practices of this five-thousand-year-old tradition, with tens of millions more nationwide." [26]

Alternative Healing: The Complete A to Z Guide to Over 160 Different Alternative Therapies states that qigong must be performed daily to accrue its many benefits. These include improved digestion, mental acuity, relaxation, physical fitness, and improved oxygen assimilation. Qigong has also been found to be effective in treating ulcers, constipation, and hypertension. [27]

Also, qigong techniques can be used to treat and heal other people. Certain qigong masters are considered to be energetic healers, who use their chi externally by directing it to strengthen the vitality of their patients.

Some external qigong masters are very powerful in their ability to move external chi. Once, when Michael was on an assignment for the Fetzer Foundation, he stopped over in Singapore for a meeting on qigong research. During his stay, he witnessed a famous external qigong master demonstrating his ability to gather and direct his chi. The Master focused his attention on a hanging bamboo birdcage on the other side of the room, over fifteen feet away. Within minutes of this master's focused concentration, the birdcage began to sway. Several minutes later, the birdcage was actually twirling around, spinning and bouncing very vigorously.

Millions of people witnessed a similar exhibition of the power of qigong on the television series "Healing and the Mind with Bill Moyers," when a qigong master, without touching the participants, was able to make these people lose their balance from a standing position. As amazing as this may seem, qigong masters in China have, for centuries, been reputed to be able to perform these stunning displays of power.

HEALTH CONDITIONS THAT RESPOND WELL TO CHINESE MEDICINE

The benefits of Chinese medicine are numerous. As stated earlier, the World Health Organization declares that acupuncture is effective in treating 104 diseases. *The American Holistic Health Association Complete Guide to Alternative Medicine* offers an overview of that vast list: "The major illnesses in each of the following categories are included [in the WHO's list]: upper respiratory tract; respiratory system; disorders of the eye; disorders of the mouth, throat, and teeth; gastrointestinal disorders; neurological and musculoskeletal disorders."[28] This overview gives you a glimpse of the scope of physical illnesses that Chinese medicine successfully treats.

However, the benefits of Chinese medicine are not limited to physical diseases and maladies. Ted Kaptchuk, author of the classic text on Chinese medicine *The Web That Has No Weaver* (Congdon & Weed, 1984), says, "In the Far East, Oriental medicine is used to encourage transformation in a wide range of situations — from splinters to catastrophic illnesses, from constipation to being spiritually 'stuck' at certain levels of samadi. The ultimate definition of the benefits the patient receives during treatment is determined within the context of the relationship of the practitioner and the patient by mutual agreement."[29] In other words, Chinese medicine can be valuable to patients in all aspects of their being.

Lisa's Story: Acupuncture Helped My Health and Saved My Business

A few years ago, I was building my own personnel business and I was meeting with failure at every turn. It wasn't long before my high stress levels showed up in my health. Looking back, I realized I hadn't slept through the night for an entire year. I had terrible, terrible migraines. My M.D. diagnosed me with asthma, which showed up as chronic coughing. Just to get through the day I had to use an inhaler six times. I was really suffering.

Several of my friends had been treated by various forms of Chinese medicine. One in particular recommended an acupuncturist that she liked. Although every penny was precious to me, I figured that going to an acupuncturist was an investment in myself. I was close to broke, but I needed energy to work. And I knew I couldn't turn my business around if I wasn't well. I felt pretty optimistic that acupuncture could help me. I figured that a billion Chinese people couldn't be wrong.

The practitioner's office was in the basement of her small home in San Francisco. It was dark and a little chilly in the waiting room. Jar after jar of 'sticks and stones' lined the walls. I guessed these were the Chinese herbs. When she ushered me into the treatment room, I was struck by how different it was from the M.D.'s offices I had been in. This room was dimly lit, pleasant feeling, and very uncluttered. There were very few items in this room besides the treatment table, a small desk, and a few books. It was very minimalist.

She asked me a few questions. She didn't speak much English. But the questions she did ask were again very different than my M.D.'s. They were well-being questions about my sleep patterns, stress levels, digestive complaints — things like that.

After I answered her questions, she motioned to me to get

onto the treatment table. I wasn't really concerned about the needles. I don't have a phobia about them and don't usually react much to pain. But what I was concerned about was the transfer of disease through the needles. I was mostly thinking of AIDS. When I heard the rustling of plastic as she removed new disposable needles from their wrappers, I quickly realized that I had nothing to worry about with this woman.

I hardly noticed the insertion of the needles. But I immediately noticed a wave of relaxation and calm throughout my body. Soon after, I fell asleep. She woke me after the treatment and I was amazed first that I had slept at all, and second that I really felt like I had rested. After I got myself off the table, she gave me a bag of herbs and instructed me on how to prepare them. Then we set another appointment.

All I knew is that I wanted to get myself home as fast as possible. I was ready for more sleep. And did I ever get it! I slept through the entire night — the first time in a year!

The next morning, I steeped my herbs in boiling water. They really smelled awful. But since I had already seen results from the treatment, I was determined to take them anyway. I know I probably shouldn't have, but I chased the herbs down with a Diet Coke. It really helped.

What happened next was nothing short of miraculous to me. During that same day, my migraines disappeared and I only had to use the inhaler once. With such great results, I was excited about continuing to work with this woman. I saw her weekly for the next three months. Over that time, I completely eliminated using the inhaler, have slept through every night since, and never had another migraine again.

Now that I am in my thirties, I realize there are things that are just a part of my life. Some of them aren't so great, like Diet Cokes. But I can count Chinese medicine as one of the good things in my life. And by the way, with all the rest I got and with my health back, I was able to turn my business around. Today it's better than I had ever imagined possible.

Applying the Five Steps to Traditional Chinese Medicine

Traditional Chinese medicine in the United States has its own issues and concerns unique from any other system of alternative medicine. In this section, you'll learn about these issues and concerns. Also, on a step-by-step basis, you'll find relevant questions and information to help you make wise choices when considering traditional Chinese medicine as a treatment option.

Additions to Step Two: Get Good Referrals

The American Association of Oriental Medicine (AAOM) provides an excellent resource service, which offers both a listing of qualified Chinese medical practitioners as well as the legal status of Chinese medicine on a state-by-state basis. They do not guarantee the work of the practitioners, but each practitioner they recommend is verified to possess either a national certification or state license, or to have had their qualifications screened by the association.

Additions to Step Three: Screen the Candidates

As you read in Step Three, there is a tremendous amount of information you can receive about a practitioner before you make an appointment. Although it is almost impossible to know if you can work well with a certain Chinese medical practitioner before you personally meet, specific, well-placed questions to the staff can help to quicken your decision and shorten your list of candidates. If the staff is not able to answer any of the following questions, save them for the personal interview with the practitioner. Here are some suggestions:

Is the practitioner certified, licensed, or registered?

Not only do the designations vary from state to state, so do the requirements for the various designations. In other words, the terms used most often to describe Chinese medical practitioners' legal status: "licensed," "certified," and "registered" are defined differently from state to state. Robert Duggan, M.Ac., Dipl.Ac., president of The Traditional Acupuncture Institute, says, "In Maryland 'registered' means they have completed a specific exam, completed required education, or have sufficient clinical experience to practice as determined by the Board Acupuncture Advisory Counsel. It is, however, very easy to find different levels of training across the country. For instance, if you were in Vermont, you could be 'registered' as an acupuncturist [Chinese medical practitioner], and start practicing even though you have no training. Ask for each state in question, what exactly does 'licensed,' 'registered,' and 'certified' mean?" [30]

The AAOM can explain the legal status of Chinese medical practitioners in your state, as well as the requirements practitioners must meet in order to legally practice.

Where did the Chinese medical practitioner study and how long was their course?

Some practicing Chinese medical providers have learned their techniques through weekend seminars that can range from one weekend to several months. Most practitioners of Chinese medicine who graduated from an accredited Chinese medical school have invested between two and four years of full-time school with thousands of hours of study to their credit. The competency and experience in Chinese medicine you receive from an accredited Chinese medical school graduate versus a weekend-trained acupuncturist is dramatic.

Also, be especially cautious of medical doctors, osteopaths, and chiropractors practicing acupuncture. In some states, M.D.'s and D.O.'s are allowed to treat with acupuncture even if they have no training. (The same is also true of chiropractors in some states.) Gail Ludwig, former executive director of the American Association of Oriental Medicine, says the AAOM considers a medical doctor who has at least six hundred hours of acupuncture training and has passed the national exam as qualified. We recommend that you do the same.

Does the practitioner treat symptoms or the causes of illnesses?

Within Oriental medicine, different types of practitioners can provide their patients with completely different results. In China, for instance, one type of practitioner would give treatments that help to eliminate uncomfortable symptoms until the patient could get to the Oriental medical doctor, who would treat the cause and, hopefully, eliminate the illness.

In this country, patients can also choose acupuncturists who just treat symptoms or practitioners of Chinese medicine who work to heal the cause of the illness. Robert Duggan says, "We have a group within acupuncture that looks at the whole body and another group that focuses on relieving symptoms. A key question for clients to answer is whether they want short-term results or long-term care." [31]

Short-term results may get you relief quickly and you may save a few dollars by reducing the number of visits to the acupuncturist. On the other hand, you may be back again soon to relieve another symptom if the cause of the first symptom was never healed.

Gail Ludwig gives an example, "If a person with shoulder pain chooses a traditional Oriental acupuncturist [Chinese medical practitioner], they may have more treatments than with an acupuncturist who just relieves symptoms. On the other hand, if that same person chose an acupuncturist who only treated symptoms, they may get immediate relief from the shoulder pain but some other symptom may appear because the *cause* of the shoulder pain was not addressed." [32]

Does the practitioner use the traditional Chinese method of acupuncture or some other style? If a different style, please explain to me what I can expect during treatment.

There are many styles of Oriental acupuncture. Some are reputed to offer a variety of experiences. For instance, the Japanese use a thinner needle than the Chinese method. Miki Shima, O.M.D., past president of the California Acupuncture Association of West Los Angeles, claims that Japanese acupuncture is pain-free. Taiwan acupuncture, however, is reputed to use more needles during treatment than the traditional Chinese technique. [33] The more you understand the dynamics of the treatments, the more of a partner you can be in the process.

How much time will the practitioner spend with me during my first visit?

If the receptionist answers, "You'll be out in twenty minutes," it is probable this practitioner is more of an acupuncturist who only treats symptoms. If the answer is an hour or more, then it is more than likely that the practitioner is trained in all the nuances of traditional Chinese medicine, which offers a more thorough examination as well as a more comprehensive approach to treatment.

Has the practitioner been successful in helping my physical complaint?

Although Chinese medicine can be effective in helping many physical problems, a cure cannot be guaranteed. On the other hand, if the practitioner has extensive experience in successfully treating your physical complaint, this practitioner may be able to help. If you are told that the practitioner will cure your problem, be very skeptical. Each person and their ability to heal are different.

Does the practitioner use disposable needles or sterilized reusable needles during an acupuncture treatment?

Sterile needles are an essential component of competent, responsible acupuncture. Illnesses can be transferred through infected acupuncture needles. According to Robert Duggan, using unclean needles in an acupuncture treatment is cause for malpractice. [34] If you have any question that the needles used at a Chinese medical practitioner's office are unclean, do not agree to treatment.

How many patients does the practitioner see per day?

If the practitioner is doing traditional Chinese medicine, they will probably see only six to twelve patients per day. If they are doing symptomatic acupuncture, then, according to Miki Shima, fifteen to twenty patients per day indicates a reasonable patient load. Some acupuncturists see many more. "The worst I've ever seen was a doctor in Taiwan who saw a hundred and fifty patients a day," Dr. Shima says. "He didn't even talk to the patient. They were all lined up. After he heard their major complaint, he just stuck needles in them." [35]

How long has the practitioner been in practice?

With experience and comprehensive training, traditional Chinese medicine is not only a technique but an effective healing art as well. It is clinical experience that provides the opportunity for mastery. An experienced practitioner may be able to provide a higher quality of care.

What is the cultural background of the practitioner?

It is possible to feel comfortable communicating with a practitioner even if you don't speak the same language. On the other hand, if you need to communicate concerns or issues that don't translate well to the Chinese perspective, you may need to see a Western practitioner of Chinese medicine. Ted Kaptchuk recommends, ". . . the more one wants to deal with one's life issues, as opposed to biophysical issues, the more important it is to be with a practitioner of your own culture. A lot of personal issues don't translate culturally. A practitioner needs to understand the cultural textures of the issue." [36] In other words, make sure you feel comfortable in your ability to communicate your needs and concerns to your practitioner.

If you are satisfied with the answers to your questions, set up a short consultation with the practitioner. A short amount of time with this practitioner should indicate to you that you can or cannot work with this professional. Be selective. Each practitioner brings his or her own styles and gifts to his practice and such qualities often must be experienced in person. Choose an acupuncturist who offers the skills as well as the relationship that will nurture your healing. The benefits may astound you.

WHAT TO EXPECT DURING A
CHINESE MEDICAL APPOINTMENT

Chinese medicine is an art as well as a series of techniques. The combination of a particular style with the individuality of the practitioner makes each session a unique experience. For this reason, no two practitioners will have sessions that are identical in every way. There are, however, some standard practices that all traditional Chinese medicine practitioners share, thus providing a glimpse of what you may experience during your treatment.

The Office Visit

In the practitioner's office, you will probably first be examined while sitting in a chair. As you describe your symptoms, the practitioner will probably observe your skin tone, skin texture, movement patterns, the strength and tone of your voice, and any body or breath odor. Most practitioners will ask copious questions covering all areas of your life. The questions can range from any emotional stress you may be experiencing to your diet to the condition of your bowel movements.

During the initial phase of the examination, the practitioner will probably perform an ancient diagnostic technique of "taking the pulses." This is done by gently pressing the radial artery of your arm at three points while reading the strength, the speed, and the rhythm of your pulse. This test is one of the cornerstones of Chinese medical diagnosis. Chinese medical practitioners claim that the basis of their ability to diagnose the condition of the major organs far exceeds in complexity and scope the information Western medical doctors obtain from taking a conventional medicine pulse reading.

Another commonly used diagnostic skill entails observing the color and texture of the tongue. In addition, some practitioners palpate or touch painful areas to find swelling or sensitivity.

Acupuncture Treatment

Your first acupuncture treatment will most likely occur after the doctor's examination and is generally performed while you lie on a table. The slim needles are inserted just below the surface of the skin by hand or through a small plastic guide. Although there are more than a thousand acupuncture points, usually no more than ten to twelve needles are inserted at a time. In most cases, the client barely feels the insertion of the needles and any discomfort disappears quickly. If it does not, the practitioner can adjust the needle so it is more comfortable.

All acupuncture needles are made of stainless steel and are hair thin. However, some styles of acupuncture use different thicknesses of needles. As we mentioned, Japanese is reputed to be the slimmest and least likely to cause discomfort. If a patient does feel the application of the needle, it is more of a pinch followed by numbness, tingling, ache, or heaviness. Sometimes practitioners use electroacupuncture or low frequency electrical stimulation. Others twirl the needle manually for extra stimulation of the chi.

Herbal Treatment

The practitioner may recommend Chinese herbs to enhance the benefits of the treatment. Herbs are given in one of three forms. The most traditional form is in "bulk." With bulk herbs, the patient is expected to brew a tea, which is ingested at a prescribed amount during the day. Other forms are powder, pills, tablets, or capsules. This option is more convenient, though its effectiveness in comparison to bulk herbs has been called into question. The third form is herbal extracts, which are placed in water and ingested. Herbal extracts are convenient for the patient, as well as easy to assimilate.

Moxibustion Treatment

This treatment is highly regarded in Chinese medicine and can be used by itself during a treatment session or in conjunction with acupuncture.

There are generally three methods of treating with moxa: as a small rolled ball placed directly on the body, as an herb twirled onto an acupuncture needle, and as a cigar-shaped stick held next to the skin. When burnt, its odor is reminiscent of marijuana, although that's where its similarity ends.

In the first method, the herb is rolled up into a small ball and placed directly on an acupuncture point or on an herb or spice, such as ginger, salt, or garlic, then lit. Moxa burns slowly and penetrates the point with heat, which further stimulates a healing response. As soon as the patient feels the moxa getting hot, it is removed.

Moxa can also be gently twisted onto an acupuncture needle that has already been inserted into an acupuncture point, then lit. The added heat, again, brings additional healing stimulation to the acupuncture point.

The last method consists of burning a processed herb, within the form of incense-like cones or cigar-shaped sticks, held just above the skin on a chosen meridian point.

COST AND INSURANCE

Cost

Traditional Chinese medicine is markedly less expensive than conventional medicine because diagnoses and remedies are provided by the practitioner during an appointment. So, in most cases, x-rays, blood tests, drugs, etc., are not necessary.

The average traditional Chinese medical treatment lasts approximately forty-five minutes and the cost averages about $45. First appointments generally take longer and are more expensive ($50 – $100). Most practitioners start patients with a program of ten treatments, if warranted, and will reevaluate progress and the need for more treatments before recommending another series. Herbs are very reasonable in cost compared to drugs. Herbs run from $10 – $50 a month.

Insurance

The coverage of Chinese medicine by insurance companies is changing rapidly, as more and more plans are beginning to cover it for certain conditions. For this reason, it is important to check with your insurance carrier to find out if they will cover Chinese medical treatments or acupuncture and, if so, exactly what they cover and for how many treatments.

However, there are also new insurance plans that cover Chinese medical treatments, while other plans are in the pilot stage for such treatments, including plans from Blue Cross of Washington and Alaska. Some of the insurance plans that cover Chinese medicine are:

Medicaid covers Chinese medicine in some states for substance and alcohol abuse.

Alternative Health Plan is available to group major medical participants nationwide. The plan covers conventional as well as alternative treatments including traditional Chinese medicine and acupuncture.

American Western Life is only available to employee group participants and covers conventional medicine, as well as many treatments and techniques of alternative medicine, including Chinese medicine. This coverage gives a flat copayment, regardless of the treatment or technique if it is within the approved three thousand credentialed providers.

American Medical Security is expanding into many states around the country. It covers acupuncture, acupressure, and prescribed herbs, as well as other alternative therapies.

CommonWell Health Plan is also currently expanding into various states. It covers Chinese medicine, as well as a wide variety of alternative health care services. This plan includes an annual wellness visit for creating goals and a personal plan for health of the mind, body, and spirit for all subscribers.

Natural Medicine Network, Inc. operates like conventional managed care networks, directing patients to approved and participating natural or holistic practitioners. Services covered include acupuncture, t'ai chi, herbs, as well as other alternative treatments.

EDUCATION, TRAINING, AND LICENSING

Over the last ten years, a strong move to standardize the education and training of practitioners of traditional Chinese medicine, as well as acupuncture, has been growing nationwide.

Unfortunately, this movement has not caught up with the licensing process, which varies widely from state to state. For this reason, as stated earlier, it is important to understand what exactly it means for a practitioner to be licensed, certified, or registered in your particular state. This information will be essential to determine if a practitioner is trained adequately to treat you.

Education and Training

Until recently, the standards for education and training in traditional Chinese medicine have varied tremendously in the United States. The Council of Colleges of Acupuncture and Oriental Medicine (CCAOM) has sought to remedy this problem by establishing standards of excellence in Oriental medical education. Over twenty-six schools now belong to this organization.

The most accepted standard for professional training is based on the credentialing requirements of the National Commission for Certification of Acupuncturists (NCCA). Generally, the NCCA certifies a student of Chinese medicine who has passed his or her exam and who has earned 1,350 hours of Chinese medical education and at least 500 hours of clinic (1,850 total hours). Ninety percent of the states that license practitioners of Chinese medicine acknowledge or use the NCCA test in their licensing practice.

On the other side of the spectrum, The American Academy of Medical Acupuncture (AAMA) recognize practicing M.D.'s and D.O.'s who have a minimum of 220 hours of training as competent to practice Chinese medicine. This assumption is highly controversial. As James Collins, of the California Acupuncture Association, writes, "Having completed medical school does not disqualify doctors to practice acupuncture. But having completed medical school does not qualify them either." [37] The critical question is whether 220 hours of training qualifies conventional medical doctors to competently practice in another system of medicine.

This controversy may soon be settled by some health insurance companies that are considering covering only Chinese medical practitioners and acupuncturists who meet the national certification standards of the NCCA.

Licensing

The laws regarding traditional Chinese medicine vary from state to state. Many states license practitioners of Chinese medicine as primary health care providers. Others permit practitioners to treat patients if the patient has been referred by a medical doctor or if the Chinese medical practitioner is under a medical doctor's supervision. In some states Chinese medicine is permitted but not regulated, while in other states Chinese medicine is actually still illegal.

The legal status of Chinese medicine in each state is monitored by the American Association of Oriental Medicine (AAOM), which also provides referrals to individual state licensing boards and Chinese medical associations who can answer specific questions about local requirements and standards.

The following is NCCA's list of states that independently license, certify, or register practitioners of Chinese medicine: Alaska, California, Colorado, Connecticut, District of Columbia, Florida, Hawaii, Iowa, Maine, Maryland, Massachusetts, Minnesota, Montana, Nevada, North Carolina, New Jersey, New Mexico, Oregon, Rhode Island, Texas, Utah, Vermont, Virginia, Washington, and Wisconsin.

States that limit acupuncture to medical doctors and osteopathic physicians: Arizona, Georgia, Indiana, Kentucky, Louisiana, Mississippi, Nebraska, West Virginia, New Hampshire, North Dakota, and Ohio.

States that limit acupuncture to medical doctors, osteopathic physicians, and chiropractors: Alabama and Illinois.

CLOSING THOUGHTS

Though you may not have previously considered using traditional Chinese medical treatments, as you can see from the information in this chapter, it may be one of the preferred treatments of choice for your condition. If, after reading this chapter you find yourself interested in exploring this alternative health care option, we encourage you to apply the processes outlined in Part I, the Five Steps, including the special additions to the Steps outlined in this chapter.

Remember that you may need a series of treatments in order to receive optimal benefits. By doing that, you will probably discover why over 25 percent of the world's population regularly use traditional Chinese medicine to meet their health care needs. ◾

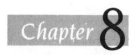

Chapter 8

NATUROPATHIC MEDICINE

Stimulating the Body's Own Power to Heal

Naturopathic medicine can reduce health costs, assist in providing primary health care to the underserved, and offer treatment for many illnesses that are not now treated effectively by existing treatments.

– U.S. Senator Claiborne Pell [1]

DID YOU KNOW THAT:

- In 1983 the World Health Organization recommended the integration of naturopathic medicine into conventional health care systems. [2]

- In 1994 Bastyr University of Natural Health Sciences, a naturopathic medical school, was awarded almost $1 million in research funds from the National Institutes of Health's Office of Alternative Medicine to research alternative therapies for patients with HIV and AIDS. [3]

- Graduates of accredited naturopathic medical colleges are required to have more hours of study in basic sciences and clinical sciences than graduates of Yale or Stanford medical schools. [4]

- The "anti-cancer" diet recognized by the National Cancer Institute was first published in a naturopathic medical textbook in the 1940s. [5]

- Graduates of accredited naturopathic medical colleges receive more formal training in therapeutic nutrition than M.D.'s, osteopathic physicians, or registered dietitians. [6]

- The government of Germany now requires conventional doctors and pharmacists to receive training in naturopathic techniques because they have been found to be so cost-effective.[7]
- Today there are over one thousand licensed practicing naturopathic physicians (N.D.'s) in the United States.[8]
- As of August 1996, twelve states in the U.S. and five provinces of Canada now license naturopathic doctors as primary-care physicians. (It is projected that all fifty states will license naturopathic physicians by the year 2010.)[9]
- Three accredited colleges educate and train naturopathic doctors in North America.[10]
- The County Council in Seattle, Washington, established the nation's first government-subsidized naturopathic medical clinic.[11]

The origin of naturopathy can be traced back to the ancient healing arts of a variety of cultures. Still, as a formal system of medicine and healing, it was developed in the United States nearly one hundred years ago by Benjamin Lust.

The Basic Principles of Naturopathic Medicine

To heal in harmony with the natural functions of the body — without harm — is the underlying principle of the naturopathic system of medicine. The intent is to support the natural healing potential of the human body as validated by modern scientific research. It is this combination of the healing power of nature and scientific methods that makes naturopathic medicine an important system of medicine for today's health care.

Naturopathic medicine's basic principles are:

1. Utilize the healing power of nature
2. First, do no harm
3. Find the cause
4. Treat the whole person
5. Preventative medicine

The American Association of Naturopathic Physicians (AANP) more fully describes these tenets as:

Utilize the Healing Power of Nature: Vis Medicatrix Naturae Nature acts powerfully through the healing mechanisms of the body and mind to maintain and restore health. Naturopathic physicians work to restore and support these inherent healing systems when they have broken down, by using methods, medicines, and techniques that are in harmony with natural processes.

First Do No Harm: Prinum Non Nocere Naturopathic physicians prefer noninvasive treatments, which minimize the risks of harmful side effects. They are trained to know which patients they can treat safely, and which ones they need to refer to other health care practitioners.

Find the Cause: Tolle Causam Every illness has an underlying cause, often an aspect of the lifestyle, diet, or habits of the individual. A naturopathic physician is trained to find and remove the underlying cause of a disease.

Treat the Whole Person: Health or disease results from a complex interaction of physical, emotional, dietary, genetic, environmental, lifestyle, and other factors. Naturopathic physicians treat the whole person, taking these factors into account.

Preventative Medicine: The naturopathic approach to health care can prevent minor illnesses from developing into more serious, chronic, or degenerative diseases. Patients are taught the principles with which to live a healthy life; by following these principles, they can prevent major illnesses. [12]

Above all, naturopathic physicians respect the natural healing power present in all systems of the human body and they attempt to focus and mobilize that power in their treatment process. N.D.'s have found that this natural healing power, if effectively mobilized, can destroy invading organisms, cast off toxins, as well as rebuild strength and vitality. Dr. Stephen Speidel, an N.D. practicing in Poulsbo, Washington, says, "A good example of how we in naturopathic medicine use the healing force in the body is what we do or don't do when a child has a fever. Often times a fever is a way that the body rids itself of a bacteria that only grows in certain temperatures.

"Most parents say, 'My God, my child has a fever. We have to stop that fever. Give him aspirin or Tylenol.' I tell them, 'Imagine that your child has a helper, which is the immune system.' If you take the aspirin, it's like taking a sledge hammer to your child's immune system and saying, 'Be quiet and sit down!' And it will. You'll win. That helper will be quiet and sit down. But your child will stay sicker longer. There are a number of studies that show antihistamines prolong the course of a cold. But if the fever or cold is allowed to run its course, the body eliminates the problem and the child gets healthy." [13]

The role of a fever as healing process may seem strange to many health care consumers who are used to using medications to eliminate its presence. Yet, many systems of healing and medicine throughout the world since ancient times have recognized the healing wisdom of letting a fever run its course.

Clearly the principles of naturopathic medicine differ significantly from conventional medicine's. In conventional medicine, relieving symptoms is the primary focus. For example, in conventional medical treatment, in the aforementioned case, the fever would be controlled or stopped by drugs. Actually in most health care situations, the elimination of symptoms is achieved through the use of drugs and, in some cases, surgery.

It may surprise some people to know that N.D.'s and M.D.'s have some areas of common ground, namely their education. M.D.'s are schooled in basic sciences and clinical sciences to prepare them for the various illnesses and emergencies they will face during their practice. N.D.'s are also well trained in all these sciences in their education. But, unlike M.D.'s, they are also trained in a variety of traditional natural therapeutics, including botanical medicine, clinical nutrition, homeopathy, acupuncture, traditional Chinese medicine, hydrotherapy, and naturopathic manipulative therapies.

N.D.'s learn how to integrate this diverse knowledge by combining their conventional medical education with the goal of providing superior health care in their practices. They weave their conventional medical knowledge with the principles of naturopathic medicine and its treatments to create a natural health care program tailored for each individual patient.

The Major Naturopathic Medical Treatments

In the past few years, naturopathic medicine has won the respect of federal and state government bodies, members of the conventional medical community, educators, celebrities, the media, and an ever-increasing number of American health care consumers. A main reason for naturopathic medicine's rise in popularity is its common-sense use of simple yet tremendously effective natural treatments. These treatments include:

Clinical Nutrition

Clinical nutrition has been one of the main cornerstones of naturopathic medicine since its inception. Studies from around the world, in a variety of medical traditions, have validated the benefits of naturopathic's nutritional principles. A vast number of documented cases of physical problems, including heart disease and diabetes, have been helped by nutrition, without unpleasant side effects or complications.

Naturopathic theory suggests that most illnesses are caused by digestive disturbances, which have led to a toxic environment in the body. As the body is overwhelmed by toxins it cannot eliminate, the health or strength of the body breaks down and symptoms of various illnesses surface. Nutritional changes are a main component to changing the diseased situation because today's processed foods and poor eating habits are the source of many of the body's toxins.

To treat chronic illnesses, many times nutritional changes are the first step toward healing in naturopathic medicine. For example, simple vegetable soups are often recommended because, as they are easy to digest and assimilate, they provide the body with vitamin and mineral nutrients without adding toxins to the body.

Hydrotherapy

If nutritional therapy is the first cornerstone of naturopathic medicine, then hydrotherapy is the second. Hydrotherapy improves digestive function by bringing additional blood (and all of its healing components) to the inner organs. The most common form of hydrotherapy is called the "constitutional," where two towels dipped in hot water, then squeezed, are placed on the front of the patient for five minutes. The hot towels are replaced with one cold towel for ten minutes. The same procedure is done on the back of the patient. During the hot portion of the hydrotherapy, the upper blood vessels are dilated while the deeper ones constrict. The cold portion of the treatment constricts the outer blood vessels but dilates the internal ones. The combination drives more blood to both the inner and outer systems, allowing the body to bring more healing nutrients to its organs and to carry away toxins.

Bernard Lust, considered the founder of naturopathic medicine, was cured of tuberculosis through hydrotherapy. According to Jared Zeff, N.D., L.Ac., former academic dean of the National College of Naturopathic Medicine, hydrotherapy is often used to treat terminal illnesses, such as cancer, as well as simple colds and infections. [14]

Dr. Zeff shares an example of how nutrition and hydrotherapy can be used together to heal an arthritic condition:

A man came to him with severe arthritis. This gentleman had artificial knees, artificial finger joints, and artificial hip joints, and he still had severe pain and swelling throughout his entire body. Dr. Zeff recommended that he eat nothing in the next week except vegetable soup (no potatoes) and to do hydrotherapy daily. Within a few days, the man's arthritis pain had greatly decreased and his swelling had decreased by 50 percent. Naturopathic physicians often find that simple dietary changes and hydrotherapy effectively treat many illnesses.

Homeopathy

Homeopathy is used by many naturopaths and is a primary treatment in their practices. Based on the "law of similars," it uses minuscule doses of naturally occurring substances to treat illness. Naturopaths have found that homeopathy fits well into their philosophical principles, since it stimulates the body's own immune system without producing unpleasant side effects. It is also documented to be effective for many illnesses, including migraines, headaches, rheumatoid arthritis, acute diarrhea, flu, and allergies.

The history of homeopathy's use spans two hundred years. Many countries embrace it as a viable healing treatment, including England, whose Royal family retains the services of a homeopath for their personal health care.

Herbs

Herbs are used by naturopathic physicians as medicine. As such, they can be extremely powerful and beneficial when used in the right dosage and in the correct combination with other herbs.

Though herbs are the main ingredient for some of the drugs used in conventional medicine, N.D.'s use herbs in a different manner than M.D.'s use them. Most drugs prescribed by M.D.'s are intended to impose an external order on the body. For example, a medicine prescribed to lower blood pressure forces the body to lower the pressure but doesn't correct the reason why the body has increased the pressure in the first place. Therefore, many patients taking blood pressure medicine as prescribed by a conventional medical doctor must continue to take blood pressure medication for the rest of their lives. Regrettably, the patient also endures the probable side effects: impotency, sexual dysfunction, and nervousness.

In contrast, an N.D.'s goal is not to impose an outside order but to correct the underlying problem. In the case of a weakened heart, an N.D. would accomplish this by using herbs that nourish and strengthen the heart, such as hawthorne berry, or herbs that disperse congestion or toxins in the body, such as dandelion root. When strengthening and detoxification occur, a patient's vitality becomes stronger, the root cause of the illness is addressed, and a permanent recovery becomes possible.

Consider the following story of a woman unable to move from the neck down: She sought the help of Dr. Zeff for an unusual type of arthritis called CNS Sjogrens Syndrome. Her symptoms included severe joint pain as well as an autoimmune lesion on the brain stem. She had the use of many of her muscles but was too weak to make them work for her. Also, her condition was irregular. One day, several months ago, she was able to walk, but for only three hours. This one fact indicated to Dr. Zeff that, unlike patients with multiple sclerosis, she didn't have nerve damage, and therefore had the possibility of recovery.

During Dr. Zeff's examination, he found that her temperature was consistently 94 degrees, which he considered to be the key to her recovery. Dr. Zeff concluded that in order for her to heal, her body temperature must go up. So he prescribed for her a combination of herbs that were warming and improved blood flow. After a couple of weeks, her temperature had risen to 96 and some days to 97 degrees. The rise in temperature has resulted in more control of her hands, greater ability to move her knees, and twice she has been able to drive her own wheelchair. Dr. Zeff's goal with this patient is to maintain a higher temperature to support her body's ability to correct the underlying causes of her condition.

Chinese Medicine

The treatments and diagnostic techniques as well as the fundamentals of Chinese medicine are a part of all naturopathic physician's training at the accredited medical colleges. (See Chapter 7 for more detail about traditional Chinese medicine.) Some naturopaths do advanced training and become licensed practitioners of Chinese medicine, using Chinese herbs, acupuncture, and acupressure in their practice.

For example, Dr. Zeff is also a licensed practitioner of Chinese medicine, and recently used acupuncture to help in a difficult case. A man came to Dr. Zeff with significant pain in his abdomen, which was the site of a "bathrobe fire" ten years before. The man had been through a number of conventional medical diagnostic regimens to find out why he was still in pain. No matter what they tried, the M.D.'s could not determine what exactly was causing his pain. Dr. Zeff talked with this man for about an hour and, from his conversation and examinations, surmised that the scarring from the burn had disrupted the flow of chi along the meridians in the area. As a result of this diagnosis, Dr. Zeff treated the man with acupuncture in order to normalize the flow of chi in the affected area.

Once the man had reclined on the treatment table, Dr. Zeff inserted five acupuncture needles, two in each foot and one in a point on the abdomen. After the insertion of the needles, the man first reported that the needle in the abdomen hurt. Then he said he felt movement and activity in the area. Then, after ten minutes, he said that he felt no pain — the first time in ten years.

The techniques of Chinese medicine can bring impressive and surprising results to many health care challenges and is considered an exceptional treatment for acute and chronic pain.

Natural Childbirth

Natural childbirth is offered by some naturopathic physicians in either a home or a clinic environment. N.D.'s are trained in natural prenatal and postnatal care involving noninvasive, nonpharmaceutical treatments. Through their treatments and techniques, N.D.'s continuously screen to make sure the mother and child are in a low-risk state. One important screening involves monitoring the mother's diet and supplements to ensure that the mother's inner nutrients are sufficient to create a healthy, normal baby. Naturopathic theory suggests that adequate nutrient levels in the mother minimize childbirth risks.

Naturopathic physicians believe counseling is an important component of their jobs as facilitators for childbirth care. Dr. Zeff says that he requires the mother and partner to invite him and his assistant to dinner. "One factor that we found that can significantly disrupt a birth is the emotional state of the mother," he says. "If, during our dinner time with the mother/couple, we notice any significant stress, then we know that counseling will be needed to minimize the mother's emotional distress so that she can relax during labor and have a normal birth." [15]

N.D.'s use many different treatments during the various stages of gestation and birth, including some that most conventional doctors are unfamiliar with. For instance, some N.D.'s use homeopathy before labor begins to help a breach baby turn to the correct "head-down" position. In some cases, the homeopathic remedy Pulsatilla is used when the baby is not yet in the right position for delivery. Naturopathic physicians have seen that within twelve hours of giving a dose of Pulsatilla to the mother, the baby turns by itself. Another remedy used by naturopathic physicians is a preparation of the herb cottonroot. This herb, usually given to the mother in tincture form, helps bring the placenta down if she has not delivered it within a normal time.

Although N.D.'s are well trained in most birthing situations, they are also quick to refer mothers to the appropriate M.D. or hospital if a risk is present that disqualifies the mother and child from a natural childbirth experience.

Counseling and Stress Management

Naturopathic physicians believe the patient's emotional and psychological makeup can greatly influence the patient's ability to heal. Therefore, they are trained in many psychological techniques, including counseling, stress management, hypnotherapy, biofeedback, and nutritional balancing.

Minor Surgery

Most people would be surprised to know that minor surgery is a part of some naturopathic physicians' practices. In addition to natural treatments of illnesses, N.D.'s are also trained to mend surface wounds; to remove unwanted foreign masses, cysts, and other superficial bodies with local anesthesia; as well as to perform circumcisions, skin lesion removal, hemorrhoid surgery, and setting of fractures.

Ayurvedic Medicine

Ayurvedic medicine is an ancient system of holistic medicine and healing from India. Its focus is on treating the whole person with diet, nutrition, and lifestyle recommendations. One of the key components of this system of healing is an appreciation of the role that one's vital energy, called "prana," plays in the healing process. Bastyr University now offers a specialization in this ancient system of medicine. As a result, some N.D.'s have earned specialty degrees in ayurvedic medicine and have incorporated it into their practices.

Physical Medicine

Naturopathic physicians use a combination of manipulative therapies, which move soft tissue as well as skeletal bones. These are collectively called naturopathic manipulative therapy and in some ways are similar to the techniques used by osteopathic physicians, chiropractors, massage therapists, and body workers in that structure is realigned to support the innate healing process of the body.

Not all naturopathic doctors use this as a major component of their practice. However, when other treatments fail to bring the desired response, then manipulative therapies can be helpful.

One gentleman who had tried a wide range of treatments to correct the weakness and pain he felt in his own right arm went to his N.D. for manipulative treatments. The N.D. found that the man had a combination of muscle spasm from stress and spinal misalignment. As a result, the nerve flow necessary for normal muscular activity was being blocked. The N.D. treated this man with manipulative therapy. The result: the gentleman felt better than he had in six months.

Misalignment of the spinal vertebrae as well as other skeletal structures can be the cause of pain or even illness in some cases. The return of vertebrae, bones, and joints to their optimal position can eliminate pain in as little as one treatment.

Jan's Story: A Friend Heals Her Psoriasis

I had just arrived for a visit at the home of Rosalynd, an ill friend. "Don't fill that prescription!" I remember her exclaiming to her husband. She had just returned from her M.D.'s office. Her voice riddled with frustration and anger, she continued, "I've got cancer! Why would I use a lotion made with a carcinogen?!?"

Rosalynd was literally fighting for her life. Yet she couldn't get a decent night's sleep because of the tremendous itching she felt from the psoriasis that covered her upper body. To relieve her discomfort from psoriasis, her M.D. had prescribed a lotion containing coal tar derivatives. Many studies had verified that these derivatives can cause cancer and Rosalynd was well aware of it. Unfortunately, the prescribed lotion was her M.D.'s best solution.

While her husband got ready for work, I calmed her down by assuring her that we certainly wouldn't call the pharmacist to fill that particular prescription and suggested that we think about another solution to her psoriasis. Then Rosalynd and I remembered a doctor she had seen before, Konrad Kail, N.D., a well-respected naturopathic physician and at that time the newly elected president of the American Association of Naturopathic Physicians (AANP). We hoped he might have a better option.

I phoned Dr. Kail and reminded him of Rosalynd's case. I described the difficulty she was having sleeping from the itching of the psoriasis and asked for his advice. He was well aware that she was battling cancer and that her immune system was compromised. He was also aware that she had chosen to work with a European M.D. whose unique chemical treatment for cancer was unfamiliar to him. Dr. Kail decided to respect Rosalynd's choice to work with her M.D. on her cancer and therefore to treat only the symptom of her psoriasis — not the underlying cause of her illnesses.

To relieve her itchy skin, he suggested a lotion that he developed that had helped many of his other patients. I asked him for a list of the ingredients, which he gladly shared with me (the main ingredient being jojoba beans). He added, "You can be sure there are no carcinogens in this lotion."

Rosalynd began using Dr. Kail's lotion. The following week she showed me that the lotion was working. I noticed that the large red scaly patches of skin on her arms and back were now smoother and a more natural color. When I asked her how she was feeling, she smiled and reported she was no longer kept awake by the terrible itching the psoriasis had caused. Three weeks later, Rosalynd proudly showed me that the psoriasis was completely gone.

I think it's possible that had Rosalynd's M.D. known of a nontoxic remedy, he would have offered it. I learned from this experience that most traditional medical schools do not teach nontoxic, noninvasive treatments. As a result, most M.D.'s are unaware of effective options like the herbal lotion prescribed by Dr. Kail. Fortunately I now know about naturopathic physicians. They are experts in nontoxic, noninvasive treatments and when I have a health care problem, I call them first.

HEALTH CONDITIONS THAT RESPOND WELL TO NATUROPATHIC MEDICINE

Naturopathic medicine is beneficial for a wide range of physical illnesses and conditions. Naturopaths claim that their ability to determine the underlying cause of the illness and to stimulate the body's own healing ability is why their medicine can be so effective where other systems of medicine are not.

One area where modern naturopathic medicine has been very effective is in the natural treatment of women's health problems. One series of clinical research studies for women suffering from cervical dysplasia (abnormal Pap smears) produced results in which of the forty-three women in the study, thirty-eight returned to normal Pap smears and normal tissue biopsy by using naturopathic medical treatments. Naturopathic medical formulas are also effectively being used as a natural alternative to hormone replacement therapy for women. [16]

An excellent example of naturopathic medical principles in action is the recent success of Dean Ornish, M.D., director of the Preventive Medicine Research Institute in Sausalito, California, in his work with heart disease. Dr. Ornish found that his patients with chronic coronary heart disease could actually reverse their conditions without drugs or surgery, a concept that before his study was not only discounted, but unheard of by the conventional medical profession. This extraordinary feat was accomplished through an extremely low-fat diet, stress reduction through meditation and yoga practices, modest exercise, and weekly participation in an emotional support group. [17]

Dr. Ornish's success validated naturopathic medicine's basic tenets and treatment approaches. Not only that, healing through nutrition, exercise, and stress management has now been recognized by many insurance companies, who reimburse for Dr. Ornish's program as an alternative to expensive and risky heart bypass surgery.

Another area where naturopathic medicine has proven to be effective is in preventative medicine and health maintenance. "I think the best position for N.D.'s is in the family practice," Dr. Kail says. "Naturopaths are the only physicians who have primary skills in health/risk analysis and disease prevention. We find that people *do* want more time with their physician, to be educated, to be given less toxic therapies. Most people are as yet unaware that naturopaths provide just those things." Kail says some of the benefits of using a naturopathic doctor are safer medicine, quicker recovery time, and, especially, prevention of future illness. "I tell my patients what they can do at home to keep themselves healthy," he says. "If we do our job right, then they don't have to see a [conventional] doctor as much. That saves money." [17]

Also, given that naturopaths are trained in natural childbirth, with their noninvasive and natural treatments, N.D.'s are able to avoid many of the complications associated with childbirth. The result is that births overseen by N.D.'s require far fewer cesarean sections than with conventional medical care.

Naturopathic medicine, although effective, does have its limitations. "The areas of expertise and efficacy of naturopathic medicine are not the same as conventional medicine," Dr. Zeff explains. "Conventional medicine excels in acute trauma care. We do not. If I were in an automobile accident, I'd want them to take me to a hospital where they can patch me up. The areas where I would not go to a naturopath are acute trauma, childbirth emergency, and orthopedic problems that require orthopedic surgery." [19]

Naturopathic medicine has been shown to be an effective approach for the treatment of ear inflammations, infections, and respiratory illnesses, as well as degenerative illnesses. Recently the National Institutes of Health took note of naturopathic medicine's success with terminal diseases and granted Bastyr University almost $1 million to research the effects of alternative therapies on HIV and AIDS patients. Leanna Standish, N.D., Ph.D., research director at Bastyr University of Natural Health Sciences and advisor to the Office of Alternative Medicine, states that initial research has found enhanced immune response and a decline in the progression of AIDS, when compared to the control study who only received conventional medical therapy. [20]

Applying the Five Steps to Naturopathic Medicine

Whether patients need help in health maintenance or a reversal of a devastating disease, naturopathic medicine is a viable option worthy of consideration. If you decide to try the skills and expertise of a naturopathic physician, use the following questions to help you make your decision.

Additions to Step Two: Get Good Referrals

The best referral source for licensed naturopathic physicians who have graduated from an accredited four-year naturopathic medical college is the American Association of Naturopathic Physicians (AANP). For a small fee, they will send you a list of qualified members who have satisfied their stringent requirements.

Additions to Step Three: Screen the Candidates

Once you have a few naturopathic physicians to investigate, call their offices and ask to speak to someone on the staff. Asking well-targeted questions can assist you in determining if this is a good doctor for you. Here are a few suggestions:

What is the doctor's educational background?

If naturopathic medicine is new to you, it would be ideal if you could work with an N.D. who has completed all the hours of study and clinical residency to graduate from one of the three accredited naturopathic colleges: Bastyr University of Natural Sciences in Seattle, Washington; National College of Naturopathic Medicine in Portland, Oregon; the Canadian College of Naturopathic Medicine in Toronto, Ontario, Canada. A fourth college, Southwest College of Naturopathic Medicine and Health Sciences in Scottsdale, Arizona, is in the accreditation process.

However, since there are only about one thousand naturopathic physicians from these medical schools practicing across the nation, it is possible that a graduate of one of these institutions will not be available to you. In that case, you will need to determine if you want to work with a respected practicing naturopath in your area who received their education and training from other sources, such as competent apprenticeship programs and other viable training.

Given that this particular group of naturopaths has not necessarily met the high standards required by the AANP, it is extremely important to use seven to ten years of full-time clinical experience as a guide when determining the competency of a naturopath who has not been formally trained at one of the accredited naturopathic medical schools.

Be very careful to thoroughly investigate N.D.'s who are not graduates of the three accredited naturopathic colleges. Not all "naturopaths" with the initials "N.D." after their name have competent training or the necessary expertise. For instance, some practitioners have been awarded Doctors of Naturopathy ("N.D.") after graduating from a mail-order school. These graduates have had possibly no clinical residency and significantly fewer hours of education, than required of graduates of the accredited naturopathic medical colleges. Training from a mail-order school is considered insufficient to legally gain licensure as an N.D. in the states that license naturopathic physicians as primary-care providers.

Knowing your practitioner is a well-trained, licensed N.D. assures a dependable level of competence. Someone who does not have that background can certainly be a risky choice and must be thoroughly investigated before beginning treatment.

Does the naturopath have experience with my condition?

Find out how many patients with your health care problem this doctor has successfully helped. The higher the number of successes by the naturopath, the better for you. Ask to talk to some of those patients. Make sure all your questions about their background, training, and expertise have been answered to your satisfaction before beginning treatment.

What is the doctor's specialty?

In most cases, in naturopathic medicine the answer to this question will be given in the types of treatment the N.D. specializes in rather than in specific physical conditions. Dr. Zeff explains, "We don't tend to specialize in systems like medical conventional doctors do, but we tend to create affinities for various therapeutic methods."[21] For instance, due to Dr. Kail's training in conventional medicine, he tends to prescribe antibiotics to avoid bacterial complications, while Dr. Jared Zeff, who is also a licensed acupuncturist, tends to use more alternative treatments.

Does the doctor use health care techniques not taught in his or her formal training at medical school? If so, what are they, what training has the doctor had in them, and how long have they used them in practice?

Naturopathic medical education includes a wide variety of alternative health care modalities, but not all. Make sure your doctor is well trained in any technique that he or she may recommend for your recovery. Check for credit hours, board certifications, and certificates of completion.

Will my insurance cover naturopathic care?

There are about seventy health insurance companies that cover naturopathic medical fees at this time. Most naturopathic offices carry a list of insurance carriers that cover naturopathic medicine and should be able to verify whether your insurance company will reimburse you for their services.

Is this N.D. licensed?

At this writing, there are twelve states that license N.D.'s as primary-care providers: Alaska, Arizona, Connecticut, Florida, Hawaii, Maine, Montana, New Hampshire, Oregon, Utah, Vermont, and Washington. It is believed that by the year 2010, all fifty states will license naturopathic physicians.

If you live in a state where N.D.'s are not yet licensed, but you would still like to work with a naturopathic physician, there are *four types* of practitioners who call themselves "naturopaths" or "N.D.'s" that you will find in an "unlicensed" state:

The first type of practitioner:

- Has graduated from an accredited naturopathic medical school
- Is a recognized member of the American Association of Naturopathic Physicians
- Is licensed to practice in one of the "licensable" states

This practitioner is qualified to see you for almost any health condition.

The second type of practitioner:

- Has not graduated from one of the accredited naturopathic medical schools
- May have received a degree or certification from a correspondence school
- Has at least seven years of clinical experience through apprenticeship with a qualified naturopath coupled with full-time personal practice

This practitioner may be qualified enough to help you. However, it is essential that you investigate their exact education and training to make sure they are competent for your needs. Jim Massey, N.D., of Portland, Oregon, admits, "Not all effective healers have initials after their names." [22]

An example of an exceptional naturopathic practitioner who does not have the "N.D." initials after her name is Yvonne Sklar of Hermosa Beach, California. Yvonne is proficient at integrating holistic health alternatives and has provided service for thousands of people worldwide over the last twenty-five years. She earned her Master Herbalist Certification from John Christopher's School of Natural Healing in Utah, and received her certification in iridology from Bernard Jensen, D.C., and is a direct protégé of his. She has also received extensive training in fasting and tissue cleansing procedures. Yvonne is currently working alongside Dr. Hans Gruenn, M.D., at his practice in Marina Del Rey, California. Her main diagnostic and treatment tools are iridology, nutrition, and herbs. The following is a story of how she helped one gentleman with psoriasis:

Yvonne Sklar's Story: Treating Severe Psoriasis

In July, 1985, I was eating at an outside cafe on the Strand in Hermosa Beach on a very hot summer day. While I was enjoying my lunch, a large robust Hawaiian man sat down at a table in front of me. It was obvious that something was amiss with him because he was fully clothed in a thick long-sleeved turtleneck shirt and long pants during a heat wave. His female friend, on the other hand, was dressed in a bathing suit top, shorts, and rollerblades.

As he settled into his chair, he pushed up his sleeves above each elbow and exposed a severe case of psoriasis that looked like lizard skin — overlapping dark scales. I realized then that he was fully clothed to hide a severe psoriasis condition which covered his entire body. My companion said, "You must give this poor man your business card. He must be in great pain." I replied that approaching him would be an intrusion of his privacy, but I secretly hoped that he would somehow find his own way to me.

Two weeks later, to my complete surprise, that same female companion of the Hawaiian man literally rolled into my office on her rollerblades. She was followed by the large Hawaiian gentleman. After introductions were made, I explained to the man that I had lived in Hawaii for many years and was familiar with the local diet (which consisted mainly of "poi," a combination of taro root, white rice, and pork). I asked the man how much poi he was eating a day. When he told me he was eating eight large bowls a day, I knew where his psoriasis came from.

I admitted to him that I had seen him on the Strand and noticed his psoriasis. I said that I guessed that it covered his body. He hung his head as if he were responsible for some crime and sadly replied, "I am in such pain. I cannot live a normal life. Can you help me?" I said, "No more poi! That's what you have on your skin!"

After I examined the irises of his eyes, I gave him the following treatment:

Herbs: Cascara Sagrada, Hops, Valarian, Scullcap, Mullein, Bayberry, Goldenseal, Juniper, Capsicum, Burdock, Comfrey, Black Walnut, Horsetail, Sage.

Supplements: Liquid Dulse, Calcium, Selica, Niacin, 2 – 4 cups of Oat Straw tea daily, carrot and celery juice with liquid chlorophyll.

Treatments: Hydrotherapy, massage and dry skin brushing; aloe vera juice — topically and orally.

Dietary Changes: no pork, no poi, lots of vegetables and fruit, a few complex carbohydrates and a little chicken.

Exercise: Moderate.

In two to three months, his skin was completely clear. He now wears shorts, sandals, and short-sleeved T-shirts. He looks like a healthy, slim Hawaiian with beautiful skin and I hear from his friends that he is happily enjoying the beach. After his skin recovered, I never saw him again. However, he has sent me dozens and dozens of patients over the years. Most recently, three good-looking construction men with bad diets! [23]

Finding a naturopathic practitioner who is not an "N.D." and yet is also well trained and experienced like Yvonne is unusual, but not impossible. Again, if you are interested in trying naturopathic medicine but do not have an N.D. in your area, ask other respected alternative providers if they know of a good naturopath. Be sure to investigate the naturopath's training thoroughly.

The third type of practitioner:
- Has not graduated from one of the accredited naturopathic medical schools
- Received his or her degree from a correspondence school
- Has not gained enough training and experience to competently treat you in naturopathic medicine

We do not recommend that you work with practitioners in this category.

The fourth type of practitioner:
- Has no formal educational training
- Has voluntarily designated him- or herself a "Naturopath" or an "N.D."
- Has little or no training to competently treat you

Working with someone in this category can be dangerous. We do not recommend practitioners in this category.

Take extra screening precautions before agreeing to treatment with any practitioners of naturopathic medicine who are not graduates of one of the three accredited naturopathic medical colleges.

Additions to Step Four: Interview the Candidate

During an interview with a naturopathic physician, find out the personal philosophy of the naturopath. "I would need to know that I could trust the doctor and if they were well trained," Dr. Zeff suggests. "I would talk to them about what their ideas are about the nature of disease, the nature of my problem, and what approach they would take to improve it. I would ask how long I could expect improvement to take and what kinds of costs are involved. The most important thing is to get a sense of who this person is, what they have to offer, as well as their credentials. You are an individual. So choose someone who fits with you." [24]

If you're looking for an N.D. who is caring and capable, you may find your search fairly easy since naturopathic physicians value the healing power that can happen in the relationship between doctor and patient. Most take the time and effort to develop a good rapport with their patients.

WHAT TO EXPECT DURING A NATUROPATHIC MEDICAL APPOINTMENT

Naturopathic physicians use specific treatment(s) that can include homeopathy, Ayurveda, and Chinese medicine, or the traditional naturopathic approach of nutrition, herbology, and hydrotherapy in their practices. These "specialties," in addition to the specific health condition of the patient, make a session with each naturopath a unique experience. However, there are some standard procedures that all naturopathic physicians use.

The Office Visit

Most N.D.'s send questionnaires to new patients that ask many personal health history questions. During a first visit, which usually lasts about an hour and a half, these questionnaires are reviewed. In addition, the N.D. will ask many lifestyle questions regarding diet, vitamin and mineral supplements taken, sleep patterns, work conditions, smoking habits, and sugar and coffee intake. In addition, some standard medical diagnostic tests are administered, such as a physical exam, and blood and urine tests.

Some naturopathic physicians also add to the first visit tests such as the Heidelberg test, which measures digestive dysfunction through gauging stomach acidity, and the urine indican test, which measures levels of toxemia.

Dr. Kail, both an N.D. and a physician's assistant, describes some differences between a visit to an M.D. and an N.D. "I found the N.D.'s do the same basic diagnosis as the M.D.'s," he says. "Naturopathic physicians go a step further and add more examinations than the typical medical doctors. For instance, digestion analysis, spinal screening, disease prevention, diet, and stress factors." [25]

Once an N.D. has made a diagnosis, the treatments prescribed will be based on the N.D.'s adherence to the fundamental principles of naturopathic medicine and to their specialty. Sometimes N.D.'s will give their patients a choice of treatments if they have a preference. "If I see a patient who has pain in his arms because his neck is out of alignment," Dr. Kail says, "I explain to them that we can do spinal adjustments, acupuncture, homeopathy, or we can do all three. Then I wait for their choice." [26]

Generally, follow-up visits with an N.D. last between thirty and forty-five minutes and involve a continuation of the treatment plan as well as an evaluation of progress.

COST AND INSURANCE

Cost

According to the American Association of Naturopathic Physicians [AANP], sessions with naturopathic physicians are about half the cost of visiting an M.D. Because naturopaths primarily rely on their own diagnostic skills, costs for extensive tests are usually minimal. This can substantially reduce the cost of naturopathic health care.

Also, naturopathic physicians are well trained in preventative medicine. Many insurance companies are realizing the long-term savings of keeping their plan members healthy. Naturopathic physicians excel at preventative medical techniques and can pass those long-term savings on to you.

Initial office visits are usually between $75 and $100 and follow-ups are in the range of $35 – $50. The prescribed supplements are usually vitamin, mineral, herbal, and/or homeopathic. Each of these supplements are far less expensive than prescriptions filled at the pharmacy. However, in the states of Arizona, Oregon, and Washington, N.D.'s are licensed to prescribe antibiotics, thyroid medicine, progesterone, as well as other drugs that may end up costing you more.

Insurance

As mentioned above, a growing number of insurance companies have recognized the value of preventative health care, a specialty of naturopathic medicine. For this reason, naturopathic medicine is being covered by more and more insurance plans. If you are fortunate enough to live in the states of Connecticut or Washington, naturopathic medical coverage is mandatory by law from all health insurance companies.

For a list of insurance carriers that cover naturopathic medicine, call the AANP or your local naturopathic physician's office. Many N.D.'s carry a list of insurance providers who cover their services.

One insurance plan that has given special attention to naturopathic coverage is American Western Life Insurance Company of Foster City, California. Their "Wellness" medical director, Marcel Hernandez, is an N.D. American Western Life provides a twenty-four-hour hot line where you can talk directly to a licensed naturopathic physician at any time, day or night. In addition, they cover all naturopathic treatments, including homeopathy, nutritional counseling, Ayurveda, massage, and physical therapy.

EDUCATION, TRAINING, AND LICENSING

Education and Training

Naturopathic physicians are well educated in the basic clinical sciences as well as natural and alternative diagnostic and treatment methods. According to the American Association of Naturopathic Physicians, "Naturopathic physicians (N.D.'s) are general practitioners trained as specialists in natural medicine. They are educated in the conventional medical sciences, but they are not orthodox medical doctors (M.D.'s). Naturopathic physicians treat disease and restore health using therapies from the sciences of clinical nutrition, herbal medicine, homeopathy, physical medicine, exercise therapy, counseling, acupuncture, natural childbirth, and hydrotherapy. They tailor these approaches to the needs of an individual patient." [27]

Graduates of accredited four-year naturopathic medical schools are justifiably proud of their education. "Essentially, naturopathic medical training is similar to conventional medical training," Dr. Zeff explains. "The first two years are virtually the same as any medical school: anatomy, physiology, microbiology, biochemistry, etc. They are taught at the same level as any other medical school. If you look at the number of hours in our classroom situation, you'll find in most cases the number of hours we spend exceeds most medical schools." He adds, "We are required fifteen hundred hours of clinical education as a minimum to graduate from the school. This is under the supervision of naturopathic doctors." [28] Medical educators and legislators have been impressed with the high standard of education required of naturopathic physicians.

Licensing

There are currently twelve states in the U.S. and five provinces in Canada that license naturopathic doctors as primary care physicians: Alaska, Arizona, Connecticut, Florida, Hawaii, Maine, Montana, New Hampshire, Oregon, Utah, Vermont, Washington, Alberta, British Columbia, Manitoba, Ontario, and Saskatchewan.

All other states in the U.S. have licensable, trained naturopaths practicing. In these states, many N.D.'s who graduated from an accredited four-year college opt to apply for licenses in other health care modalities, such as acupuncture or chiropractic, in order to stay protected by law. Others choose to practice without protection of the law. In most states, naturopathic medicine is "alegal" (neither "legal" nor "illegal"). In these states, naturopathic medicine is neither protected nor regulated. Regrettably, this can be somewhat confusing for the health care consumer.

Jim Massey, N.D., says, "When I was in North Carolina, there must have been thirty people practicing as N.D.'s. Only four of them had been to four-year medical schools. You could pay $25 and set up a tax I.D. number and start practicing immediately. You'd have to kill somebody before they'd come after you for practicing without a license. It isn't fair to the public to be duped by these people with the phony initials after their names." [29]

Again, to protect yourself and your health, call the American Association of Naturopathic Physicians. They represent the largest contingency of licensed naturopathic physicians who have graduated from an accredited school.

CLOSING THOUGHTS

Licensed naturopathic physicians are filling an important need as primary health care providers who are experts in nontoxic, noninvasive treatments. As highly skilled and well educated about the human body as graduates of Stanford or Yale medical schools, they bring the best of ancient natural treatments and scientific research to their medicine. Naturopathic medicine could serve you as well as the growing number of Americans who are calling their naturopathic physician first for their health care needs.

Chapter 9

CHIROPRACTIC MEDICINE

Healing the Body with Nerve Innervation

The core of chiropractic is that most important concept: the belief in the body's inherent ability to heal itself by reestablishing an unobstructed flow of nerve impulses between the brain and the rest of the body.

— Dean Bender, D.C.

DID YOU KNOW THAT:

- The forty-five thousand practicing chiropractors make up the second largest group of primary-care providers in the United States. [1]

- Between 12 and 15 percent of Americans are under the care of a chiropractic doctor. [2]

- According to the Utah Study from the *Journal of Occupational Medicine* in 3,062 cases of injured workers, chiropractic care was 73 percent more effective than medical care and cost 67 percent less. [3]

- Thirty percent of Americans have used chiropractic and ninety percent stated that treatment was effective. [4]

- By 1993, Americans were spending $3.3 billion annually on chiropractic care. [5]

- There are seventy colleges of chiropractic graduating approximately two thousand trained chiropractors a year in the U.S. [6]

The growth of chiropractic as a profession has been one of medical protest involving a turbulent social history. Since the profession's inception, struggles against the medical establishment for legitimacy as well as conflicts within its own ranks have occurred. Historically, chiropractic is considered an American heritage. "The rise of chiropractic," wrote British medical historian Brian Inglis, the author of the *History of Medicine*, "has been one of the most remarkable social phenomena in American history . . . yet has gone virtually unexplored." [7] Still, its success as an alternative health care system has brought it legitimacy and acceptance by both the government and the public.

The Basic Principles of Chiropractic Medicine

Today, chiropractic is recognized in all fifty states as well as the District of Columbia. Chiropractors are now found in most countries of the Western world, and tens of millions of people use chiropractic as primary providers of health care. Still, many people are largely uninformed about what chiropractic health care involves and just what a chiropractor does. The "Chantilly Report" to the National Institutes of Health identifies four major principles of chiropractic medicine:

1. The human body has an innate self-healing ability and seeks to maintain homeostasis or balance.
2. The nervous system is highly developed in humans and influences all other systems in the body, thereby playing a significant role in health and disease.
3. The presence of joint dysfunction and subluxation [misalignment of joints] may interfere with the ability of the neuromusculoskeletal system to act efficiently and may lead to or be a cause of disease.
4. Treatment is based on the chiropractic physician's ability to diagnose and treat existing pathologies and dysfunctions by appropriate manual and physiological procedures. [8]

In other words, the main principle of chiropractic medicine theorizes that the functions of the body are controlled by the nervous system. Given that the nervous system is surrounded and intertwined within the musculoskeletal system, any distortion of the structure of the musculoskeletal system will impact the nervous system, including the end destination of the nerve — whether it is a muscle for motion, a joint, an area of skin sensitivity, or an organ for function. Chiropractic counteracts the effects of poor posture, insufficient muscle tone, injury, and stress that can cause the musculoskeletal structure to be out of alignment. The goal of chiropractic treatment is to return that structure to proper alignment and balance so that the entire body can function efficiently. This is achieved primarily through manipulation of the articular joints and other related treatments.

"Most people assume that since we work with the nervous system through the back, that we are only 'back doctors.' That isn't the whole picture," says Stuart Garber, D.C., D. Hom. (MED.)[9] "Chiropractors are nerve doctors, and therefore whole body doctors. For instance, if there is a structural imbalance, then somewhere in the body there is also a functional imbalance. Chiropractic can be the answer to correcting these functional imbalances too." Dr. Garber adds, "A chiropractor's job is to allow the body to fully express itself by removing obstacles, in the form of structural imbalances, from the nervous system's ability to control the body's functions. For this reason, chiropractic medicine is used to treat a variety of illnesses and ailments as well as to enhance overall health and well-being."[10]

The Philosophical Controversy: Straights or Mixers

Today, not all chiropractors practice the same philosophy of chiropractic treatment or use the same techniques in treating their patients. This disparity of ideology and treatment approach fuels a heated debate that splits the chiropractic profession into two distinctive schools of thought. These two schools are often described within the chiropractic community as the "straights" (also known as "conservatives") and the "mixers" (also known as "liberals").

The "straight" chiropractors consider themselves to be

technicians of pure chiropractic theory. The straights generally limit their practice to manual manipulation of the spine and for this reason view chiropractic as a limited healing art. Their main focus is on correcting subluxation in order to improve health. (Subluxation is a misalignment of two bones, usually vertebrae of the spine, at the joint that connects them.) They believe that the innate healing ability of the body is accelerated by chiropractic manipulation so they do not need to use other techniques. They use x-rays as a major diagnostic tool to assess misalignment of the skeletal structure. Also, they confine their examination to chiropractic purposes, excluding medical diagnostic testing or giving medical advice to patients. Straights make up approximately 15 percent of the practicing chiropractors in the United States.

"Mixer" chiropractors are noted for using more diagnostic and health care techniques. Their practice of chiropractic is more comprehensive in scope, with many applying holistic principles in their approach to treatment. For example, they use x-rays to diagnose not only misalignment, but also other illnesses. Mixer chiropractic schools train their students to be competent in general diagnosis, including training in such diagnostic techniques as magnetic resonance imaging, laboratory tests analysis, and CAT scans, in addition to chiropractic diagnostic procedures used by straights. Mixers are also more thoroughly trained in nutrition, exercise therapy, and lifestyle analysis than straights. In addition, many mixer chiropractors continue their education and earn diplomates (a graduate degree) in specialties such as nutrition, sports medicine, radiology, pediatrics, or orthopediatrics. They may also be trained in other manual or mechanical techniques and diagnostics not always offered in chiropractic schools, such as craniopathy, applied kinesiology, vector point therapy, sacro-occipital technique, activator technique, and bio-electrical therapy.

We know of several excellent mixer chiropractors who have very different focuses in their practices. For instance, Robin Mayfield, D.C., Diplomate Acupuncture, not only is a licensed chiropractor, but also has post-graduate training in acupuncture. So a session with Dr. Mayfield might include the use of acupuncture to support healing of a specific condition as well as homeopathic remedies to take as supplements in between office visits. Another excellent chiropractor, Dean Raffelock, D.C., Diplomate, International Board of Applied Kinesiology, and certified acupuncturist, uses his expertise learned in his graduate degree in Applied Kinesiology (AK), a diagnostic technique which uses muscle testing to evaluate muscular as well as organ system strength. A session with Dr. Raffelock would probably include a variety of diagnostic and treatment methods, including AK and Chinese pulse and tongue diagnosis to determine muscle and organ weakness and to test the effectiveness of specific nutrients, and herbs to correct any imbalances found by the tests.

As in any philosophical battle, each side has its criticisms of the other. According to Thom A. Gelardi, D.C., president of Sherman College of Straight Chiropractic, "Students and graduates of CCE [Council on Chiropractic Education — mixer] colleges must put up with the frustration of having assumed an unlimited medical objective on the one hand and being severely limited in the education, tools, technology, and legislative authority necessary to fulfill the objective on the other. CCE colleges are guided by the medical mission, i.e., to prepare students to treat disease. SCASA [Straight Chiropractic Academic Standards Association] colleges are guided by the chiropractic mission, i.e., to train practitioners to correct subluxation [misaligned vertebrae and joints]." [11]

Alan H. Adams, D.C., professor and vice president for professional affairs at the Los Angeles Chiropractic College, states, "In case and practice laws [straight] chiropractors are seen as having ethical problems in terms of the doctor's responsibility to the patient. The first responsibility is to determine what is wrong with the patient and then to determine if chiropractic care is appropriate. If not so, then refer the patient to appropriate health care. Straight chiropractors don't see their role as diagnosing what is wrong with the patient, they see themselves as just determining spinal dysfunction and spinal subluxation." [12]

These philosophical differences can result in a substantial difference in the comprehensiveness of the care a patient receives. Straight chiropractors may have an advantage if you wish to focus on problems related strictly to spinal and skeletal misalignment. But don't expect them to diagnose and treat other maladies. On the other hand, mixer chiropractors can diagnose and treat a wide range of diseases and illnesses, but you should make sure that they have the specific training and qualifications to do so. Whichever type of chiropractic you prefer, it is important that you find a chiropractor who not only has your best interest at heart, but is also qualified to work with you and sensitive enough to recognize when to refer you to another health care provider.

The Major Treatments of Chiropractic Medicine

The following are the major treatments used by both "straight" and "mixer" chiropractors:

Chiropractic Manipulation

Although spinal manipulation, the primary treatment used in chiropractic medicine, has been used since Hippocrates' time to treat back pain, the system of chiropractic medicine was founded by Daniel David Palmer in the U.S. in the 1890s. Palmer used his knowledge of spinal therapeutics, anatomy, physiology, the nervous system, and magnetic healing to create a new healing theory that linked illness with the misalignment of the vertebrae.

Chiropractic health care most often uses a technique called "chiropractic manipulation," more often referred to as an "adjustment," to help put the musculoskeletal system in balance. A chiropractor will, with his or her hands, apply pressure to a vertebrae or other misaligned joint of the body. The pressure is applied so that the vertebrae or joint is returned to its optimal position. When that occurs, most times patients hear a popping noise, similar to a "cracking of a knuckle." Most people feel an immediate release and ensuing relaxation in that area as the muscles and other soft tissue normalize, and as blood and nerve flow increase.

A colleague of ours had a personal experience with the benefits of chiropractic manipulation. Alan was in a biking accident in which he was thrown twenty feet in the air onto a dirt road. Other than minor scrapes and bruises, he did not believe anything was wrong with him. Alan was surprised to find a week later that his left hand was not able to grasp small objects. This became crystal clear to him when he attempted to pick up his keys and his hand could not hold them. When Alan went to see his chiropractor, he learned that not only had he sprained his shoulder, but that several vertebrae in his neck were out of alignment. First, the chiropractor taped his shoulder to avoid further injury. Then he performed a chiropractic manipulation on his neck. There was a loud popping sound and almost immediately the use of his hand returned. He never had a problem with it again.

Spinal manipulation is an excellent medical treatment because, in many cases, it can bring quick relief to a painful musculoskeletal condition.

Physiotherapeutic Treatments Used by Both Schools of Chiropractic

These are external treatments that help relax the muscle tension of the patient so the chiropractor can make a manual correction of a subluxation and/or support the healing of the body, keeping the musculoskeletal system in its optimal position.

Heat Therapy — Just as a warm bath can soothe tense muscles, chiropractors use a variety of heat sources to relieve pain, improve circulation, and promote healing. Some of the methods they employ are electro/mechanical devices, including ultrasound, radiant devices (shortwave diathermy), microwave, infrared and ultraviolet radiation, hot packs, and hot baths.

Cold Therapy — Most people know the wisdom of "icing" a sprain or other muscle injuries. Chiropractors use this same wisdom to mobilize the many healing properties of cold with the application of ice, ice packs, or ice massage. Cold therapy is used to reduce circulation, reduce swelling, and to reduce or eliminate pain.

Immobilizing Therapies limit or completely stop the motion around injured joints by mechanical and nonmechanical devices. Techniques used to do this include casting, bracing, wrapping, and splinting.

Traction stretches the spine and relieves strain on a subluxation.

Chiropractors also use first-aid treatments for patient injuries if required as an adjunct to their other skills.

"Mixer" Physiotherapeutic Treatments

There are a number of additional techniques used by mixer chiropractors. These involve therapeutic treatments for the musculoskeletal system, which use tools such as water and electrical stimulation devices to speed the recovery of injuries and illnesses. These include:

Hydrotherapy is the application of water in a variety of therapeutic manners, including underwater exercise, whirlpool baths, heated baths, and soaking. These techniques massage injured or tense parts of the body to increase circulation and reduce the stress of physical therapy.

Recently a colleague of ours had minor surgery and prematurely used some already stressed muscles. The result: Her back muscles went into severe spasms that made it difficult for her to move around. She got into a lukewarm Jacuzzi with jets pointed at her stressed muscles and felt some welcome relief.

Electrotherapy is the application of electro-stimulation to stimulate and/or exercise muscles, to help eliminate the collection of body fluids, or to increase circulation.

Several years ago, a close friend of ours, Gena, was in an

automobile accident. During the impact, her head was thrown back and forth, causing "whiplash" on her neck and upper back. Her chiropractor, Fred Lerner, D.C., Ph.D., F.A.C.O., had helped develop the microcurrent unit and used it in his practice. Before adjusting Gena's neck and back, Dr. Lerner placed pads of electrodes attached to the unit on the insertion points of her injured muscles. When he turned on the machine, the electrical stimulation felt like a mini-massage on her muscles. After twenty minutes of this treatment, Gena's aching muscles were more relaxed so Dr. Lerner could more easily and quickly adjust her vertebrae to their correct position.

Ultrasound converts electricity into sound waves that create a micro-massage to disperse fluids, reduce swelling, increase circulation, and relieve spasms. This treatment is very helpful in treating tendinitis, frozen shoulder, and bursitis.

Other Treatments Used by Mixers

Vitamin and Mineral Supplements are used to address deficiencies that may promote or cause certain types of dysfunction of the nervous system and other organ systems in the body.

Nutritional pioneer Bernard Jensen, D.C., Ph.D., recommends manganese supplements to patients whose spinal manipulations do not stay in place. Since the joints themselves have a large percentage of manganese in their makeup, he surmised that a lack of manganese in the overall system would weaken the joint's ability to "hold" the bone. In Dr. Jensen's opinion, the ingestion of manganese would help to reverse that condition. [13]

Nutrition and Diet — Often, a sound nutritional program is used as an adjunct therapy to support the health of the patient. If the body is fed with food that is low in the vitamins and minerals needed to strengthen or repair the musculoskeletal system as well as other systems, its ability to heal itself is compromised. As a result, many chiropractors place great importance on the diet and nutrition of their patients.

For example, some chiropractors suggest that their patients eliminate certain foods (high fat, salty, overly processed) and incorporate more high-nutrient foods such as fresh vegetables, fruits, and grains. Eating these foods promotes physical strength, health and vitality, and makes a chiropractor's job easier.

Physical Therapy utilizes exercises that can be performed actively by the patient or by a therapist on the patient. The exercises increase muscle tone, improve flexibility, improve circulation of blood and lymphs, and can prevent adhesions and fixations of joint surfaces.

Sacro-Occipital Technique (SOT) places special focus on the relationship between the cranial bones (bones of the skull) and the sacro-pelvic bones (bones of the pelvis and lower back). The theory is that any subluxation of the spine is compensation for the imbalance of either or both the cranium and the sacrum. Therefore the cranium and sacrum are adjusted first. Other subluxations that don't balance themselves naturally from this process are then adjusted.

Craniopathy is a technique that focuses on the bones of the skull and the spinal fluid, which moves in pulse-like waves through the skull and the rest of the spinal structure. If the practitioner feels a subtle obstacle while feeling the pulse of the spinal fluid, the cranial bones are gently adjusted to eliminate the obstruction and to bring that entire system into balance.

Activator Technique is an adjustment technique that involves the use of a small hand-held, rubber-tipped instrument called an "activator." This instrument gently and painlessly moves vertebrae. This technique can be used in addition to or in place of manual adjustments. Its results are essentially the same: moving vertebrae to their optimal position. However, the activator technique is sometimes called "nonforce adjustment" because it is gentler than a manual manipulation.

Applied Kinesiology is a diagnostic technique based on the theory that complementary muscles can indicate the strength or weakness of the other muscle as well as corresponding organ systems and glands. By testing the strength of one point, a trained AK practitioner can determine if its corresponding point, whether another muscle or organ, is in a stregthened or weakened state. This technique allows AK practitioners to test entire muscle and organ systems as well as to test whether a supplement is effective and at what dosage. Some advanced practitioners of AK claim they can even test for the presence, type, and location of bacteria, viruses, and parasites.

Network Chiropractic combines conventional mechanical or structural chiropractic approaches with biofield (energy field) approaches to evaluate and correct abnormalities of the spine and nervous system. It involves the use of various chiropractic techniques in specific sequences depending on the degree and type of subluxation. Donald Epstein, D.C., originator of network chiropractic, states, "This is different than attempting to match the vertebrae being adjusted to a specific technique. The difference lies in the sequence of the adjustments and the 'networking' of the various methods." [14]

Amy's Story: No Neurosurgery for My Baby

We planned my daughter's birth to be at home. When Ivy Rose finally arrived, she was two weeks late and her birth was very difficult. Her head was turned so that she couldn't easily move through the birth canal. When she was finally born, her face was very bruised, her head wasn't symmetrical, her right eye was recessed very far back compared to her left eye, and her ears were not evenly lined up.

I shared my concern with our midwife about the abnormal shape of Ivy's head. The midwife told me that as long as Ivy's soft spot was still soft, her cranial bones could adjust themselves. So I waited and I watched.

In the meantime, Ivy's right eye began to develop a thick discharge that became very crusty. Not only that, she developed a bad case of thrush. I was becoming more and more concerned that something needed to be done. From three to six weeks of age she just cried constantly.

I realized I needed to take action. Her head was still asymmetrical and there was no indication that this condition was improving naturally so I took Ivy to Children's Hospital. There a nurse at the pediatric department referred me to a neurosurgeon, after telling me that my baby would probably need surgery!

Before Amy could see the neurosurgeon, I found and bought a book entitled, *Baby Beautiful: A Handbook of Baby Head Shaping*. From reading this book I came to realize that many babies have problems with irregularly shaped heads, especially after a difficult birth. The book was full of stories and techniques on how to help a baby develop a normally shaped head. I didn't feel comfortable trying these techniques on Ivy Rose by myself, but I realized that there must be some kind of professional who can do this for her.

Fortunately, at this time my husband was teaching a martial arts seminar and many of the participants, who had come from around the country, were massage therapists. My husband shared Ivy Rose's condition with one lady who knew a lot about body work techniques. She said she would explore our community and find a professional who could help our baby. This is how we came to Dr. Robin Mayfield.

We placed a call to Dr. Mayfield and explained the situation and she told us to come immediately to her office. After Dr. Mayfield tenderly and thoroughly examined Ivy Rose, she explained that some of Ivy Rose's cranial bones were on top of each other while others were jammed together. That was causing the misshaping of her head and probably the other problems she was having. Dr. Mayfield did some very gentle spinal manipulations on Ivy's neck and back. She did what she called craniopathy, or cranial adjustments — very gentle and subtle adjustments to

Ivy's cranial bones. I could tell something significant was changing in Ivy Rose's head because Ivy had this stunned look on her face. But she seemed to be okay.

After the first session, I could see some small changes in the shape of Ivy's head. Dr. Mayfield said she needed to work slowly and that we should bring Ivy Rose back once a week for a few months. Then she gave me some homeopathic remedies to help heal the discharge from Ivy's eye as well as for the thrush. Three-and-a-half weeks after we started working with Dr. Mayfield, the discharge from Ivy's right eye had disappeared and so had the thrush.

After two months, Ivy looked so much better! Her right eye looked normal on her face. Her head was almost completely symmetrical and her ears were evenly placed on her head. She really looks beautiful now! I'm so grateful to have found someone who could help Ivy without having to do the surgery the pediatric nurse felt was required. I know Ivy Rose is going to be fine now.

HEALTH CONDITIONS THAT RESPOND BEST TO CHIROPRACTIC MEDICINE

The most documented benefit of chiropractic medicine is for relief of lower back pain. One study conducted by the Rand Corporation, a leading think tank and research firm, found that "spinal manipulation is the most commonly used conservative treatment for back pain and is supported by the most research evidence of effectiveness in terms of early results and long-term effectiveness." [15] In addition, other studies in the U.S. and abroad have indicated that chiropractic techniques are both effective and cost effective in treating lower back pain. *The British Medical Journal*, for example, compared chiropractic and hospital outpatient management of patients with acute and chronic mechanical lower back pain. They found that chiropractic treatment was significantly more effective, particularly with patients with chronic and severe lower back pain. [16]

Dr. Raffelock shares a personal story of how chiropractic not only relieved his father of a painful lower back condition, but also inspired him to pursue a career:

Dr. Raffelock's Story

When I was about eight years old, my father was suddenly unable to stand up or walk. It was a curious feeling to see my father, a man who seemed to me all-powerful, to be incapable of executing the most basic movements. I remember feeling confused by this and a little afraid.

The doorbell rang. I was really surprised to see Herman at my house. Herman was a man who lived down the street from us. We didn't see much of him. He really kept to himself. But I knew him because I rode my bike every day past his garden and it was a great garden.

Curious as to why he was there and what would happen next, I followed him and my mother up to the bedroom where my father was lying. There I saw Herman twist and pull a little on my father's back, hip, and neck. Then, almost as soon as Herman was finished, I was astounded to see my father get up and walk as if he hadn't been in any pain at all that morning. It was nothing short of a miracle to me. First my father was completely unable to move and then he was fine. I was amazed!

I trailed my father to the bathroom with a million questions about what had just occurred. He answered a few of them to his best ability. Soon after, I announced to my father with great certainty that I was going to be a chiropractor when I grew up so I could fix people too. He leveled his finger at me and said, "Deanie, you're going to be a real doctor when you grow up, not a chiropractor." I was a little perplexed by this.

I watched Herman walk down the stairs. My mother opened the door and thanked him. As he turned to leave our home, he took a moment, and looked at me. Then he smiled broadly and winked.

Some years later when I was choosing a career, I seriously considered my father's hope that I become a physician. But I couldn't forget Herman and the miracle he brought into our home that day so many years before. It wasn't long before I just knew. I was going to be a chiropractor.

There are numerous studies that have proven the benefit of chiropractic medical treatments for many other conditions. For example, according to the *American Holistic Health Association's Complete Guide to Alternative Medicine*, "A study is being conducted that compares the outcomes of medical treatment and chiropractic treatment [in middle ear infections for children]. While it is not complete, preliminary findings suggest that the chiropractic adjustment seems to have a significant beneficial effect." [17]

Also, the *Journal of Manipulative and Physiological Therapeutics* reported the findings of a study done at the National College of Chiropractic in Lombard, Illinois, which indicated that the subluxation of the spine may cause the stress response on a chronic basis in the body and therefore result in suppressed immune performance. On the other hand, a chiropractic adjustment that corrects spinal subluxation can reverse the stress response and increase immune performance. [18]

Chiropractic has also been shown to be an effective treatment in alleviating or eliminating headaches and migraines. A study in the *American Chiropractic Association Journal of Chiropractic*, entitled "Wight Study on Recurring Headaches," reported that almost 75 percent of patients with recurring headaches and migraines were either cured or experienced reduced headache pain after receiving chiropractic manipulations. [19]

More and more, chiropractic continues to prove itself to not only be an effective treatment for a wide range of health conditions, but also a cost-effective, efficient system of medicine at the same time.

Applying the Five Steps to Chiropractic Medicine

If you are looking for a good chiropractor for your health care, having a basic understanding of the chiropractic principles and treatments will help you make an educated choice. But there is more to a good chiropractor than just a quick adjustment. You'll want to find a chiropractor with the expertise and personal characteristics that match your needs. In order to do this effectively, the following information and recommended additions to the Five Steps are provided.

Additions to Step Two: Get Good Referrals

Your first step in finding a chiropractor is to find candidates who are licensed and trained. Two chiropractic associations can help you to do that.

The International Chiropractor's Association (ICA) can supply you with a list of licensed members of their association who practice in your area. Members must be graduates of an accredited chiropractic college and eligible to sit for licensure in their individual states. Both straight and mixer chiropractors are members, but membership predominately consists of straight chiropractors.

The American Chiropractic Association (ACA) offers a similar list of licensed chiropractors in your area. Their members must be graduates of CCE-accredited colleges and licensed by their states. The exact proportion of mixer chiropractors to straight chiropractors is unclear, but mixers form the majority in this association.

Additions to Step Three: Screen the Candidates

Once you have a few chiropractors to investigate, call the office of each one and speak with a staff member. The answers the staff member gives you to a few well-thought-out questions will quickly tell you if this chiropractor can meet your needs and standards. As you talk to the staff, ascertain how helpful they are. "In chiropractic we are providing a consumer service," Dr. Stuart Garber, D. Hom., says. "Even when interested people call, they should feel that the staff is genuinely interested in them."[20] To determine whether you think this chiropractor might be right for you, we suggest you ask the following questions:

Does the chiropractor practice straight or mixed chiropractic care?

Most staff members should be aware of this distinction and provide you with a direct answer. If by chance they don't, ask if the chiropractor uses other treatments besides chiropractic manipulation.

Does the doctor use techniques or treatments not taught in chiropractic medical college. If so, please describe what they are, how can they help me, the doctor's training in those techniques, and how long has he or she has used them in practice?

There are some exceptional techniques chiropractors can learn in seminars and workshops that are not offered in chiropractic college. During your investigation, make sure that the doctor is well trained in any of these techniques or treatments. Listen for certificates of completion and credit hours. If the doctor has included treatments from a different system of medicine, such as acupuncture, be certain the doctor is board certified and qualified.

How often does the doctor attend additional chiropractic and other health care education?

In order to renew chiropractic licenses, D.C.'s must attend a certain amount of additional hours of education. A doctor who attends classes above the requirement is better equipped to keep up with the advancements within his or her profession and provide quality care to you.

How long is a typical first visit with the doctor?

If the staff answers that you'll be out in twenty minutes, be cautious. There are chiropractic "mills" where doctors see up to one hundred patients a day. Under those circumstances, you will not get the best care. Dr. Fred Lerner, an expert witness in chiropractic malpractice cases, explains, "It's not so much the technique that indicates malpractice, it's the quality of the care delivered to the patient, how thorough they were in taking a complete history and in making a responsible diagnosis." [21]

Making a competent diagnosis in twenty minutes may be possible but is the rare exception. Most good chiropractors schedule forty-five minutes to one-and-a-half hours for a first visit.

Does the doctor require all patients to have x-rays?

If so, it's important that you determine why. "A lot of chiropractors are being told to x-ray all patients as a way of protecting themselves," Dr. Lerner says. "For example, if a patient is adjusted and has a rare tumor in a bone and the bone fractures as a result of an adjustment, the doctor would probably be sued for negligence because he [or she] didn't x-ray the part first."[22] Some chiropractors, though, x-ray to check spinal malalignments instead of taking the time to examine you. This can not only cost you money, but also expose you to unnecessary radiation. Ask if the chiropractor would be willing to limit x-rays to the initial physical exam and repeat them only if follow-up exams warrant them.

Additions to Step Four: Interview the Provider

If the answers to your questions encourage you to pursue this chiropractor, set up a short consultation with this doctor. Don't be shy about asking the chiropractor questions. Within a short amount of time you should be able to get a sense of whether you and this doctor can work together. Make sure that you are confident in his or her skills as well as the doctor's commitment and willingness to provide you with the best care. "Interview your doctor," Dr. Lerner recommends. "Don't be afraid to check them out. You have to understand, you are going to entrust your life to this person. You better believe that if I were entrusting my life to their advice, I'd want to know where they are from, what they do, what they know, how they work, and how long they have been doing their work."[23]

How do you determine the necessity and the frequency of treatments?

Determining how many chiropractic treatments are reasonable can be tricky. Historically chiropractors have been taught to treat three times a week for four weeks, twice a week for four weeks, once a week for four weeks and then place the patient on "maintenance care" as needed. More recently, the trend is toward outcomes of care and regular evaluation of how the patient is healing — not to a prescribed number of treatments.

How will we know that the treatment is working?

If you are not getting the results you'd like within the time period you'd like, it is sometimes difficult to determine when to stop treatment. "Our problem is that people feel better differently," Dr. Garber says. "Some people feel better almost immediately even if the problem is not fixed. Those are the people who are hard to keep in your office. Many times, though, when the symptoms are gone the body is still healing. Then there are other people who don't get symptomatic relief until everything falls into place. Then all of a sudden, they feel better." [24] Given this, it is important to keep good lines of communication with your doctor. Listen to their observations about your progress and prognosis and balance that with your own observations and intuition.

WHAT TO EXPECT DURING A CHIROPRACTIC APPOINTMENT

A visit to the chiropractor is both similar to and distinctly different from a typical visit to a conventional medical doctor. As a new patient, you should expect to provide a medical history as well as details about your present condition. Also, you will probably undergo a clinical examination that at a minimum would include your vital signs, height, weight, blood pressure, and pulse rate. After that, expect the exam to focus on your current symptoms. The chiropractor may be interested in your ability to walk, bend, and sit up. The doctor may do a posture analysis to find any muscular imbalance or curvature of the spine. Further, he or she might also measure your range of joint motion, both actively and passively.

Probably the biggest difference you will notice with a chiropractor is that the chiropractor will "palpate," or touch, the spine, trying to find any areas of swelling or fluid retention, if areas of the spine are hot or warm, how the spinal joints move, and if there are any muscle spasms. The doctor might try to measure the spinal temperature, which shows changes in the sympathetic nervous system and its activity.

If your muscles are especially tight, the chiropractor may use heat or an electrical device to help relax your muscles. This enables the chiropractor to easily align your spinal vertebrae without undo discomfort to you.

During your session, the doctor will probably perform a chiropractic manipulation to misaligned vertebrae. To begin, the doctor may position you on a chiropractic table or have you sitting up in a chair. Then the doctor will push on your spine, upper back or hip, or twist your neck gently. Again, you may hear a "popping" noise as the chiropractor completes this treatment. This indicates that the joint has been replaced to its correct position. "Chiropractic is a very physical treatment," Dr. Garber says. "Each chiropractor's touch is different, but the manipulations should feel smooth." [25] In most cases, a patient should feel some degree of relief from the symptoms immediately after the treatment.

Depending on the philosophy of the chiropractor, as well as his or her advanced training, the doctor may suggest nutritional analysis, vitamin or mineral supplements, homeopathy, acupuncture, or deep tissue massage. Usually the chiropractor will then suggest when and how often you should return to accomplish the agreed upon health care goal.

COST AND INSURANCE

Cost

There is a great disparity of fees charged among chiropractors. An initial office visit can cost as little as $30 or as high as $300 or more. Fortunately the majority of chiropractors charge fees on the lower end of this scale. High fees do not guarantee a quality chiropractor, nor does low cost imply an inferior chiropractor. Given this, it is extremely important to determine for yourself what price seems fair to you for the services rendered.

In addition, you may be asked to pay for supplements, vitamins, foods for a special diet, or even an electrical stimulation device for muscular relaxation. These additional charges can quickly add up in some offices. The range of cost of supplements per visit can run from as little as $10 to as much as $200 or more. Again, as recommended in Step Three: Screen the Candidates, we recommend that you ask a staff member *before* your appointment about the cost for a typical first visit, including supplements.

Most initial chiropractic visits, however, take from forty-five minutes to seventy-five minutes and generally cost from $50 – $150. Subsequent visits cost less at $20 – $50 and last fifteen to thirty minutes.

Insurance

Seventy-five percent of all insurance companies, including Medicare, now cover chiropractic treatments. In addition, worker's compensation plans in all states cover chiropractic care. The key, again, is whether an insurance company will consider your chiropractic care medically necessary. Find out from your insurance carrier their policy for coverage and reimbursement of chiropractic care.

EDUCATION, TRAINING, AND LICENSING

Today's chiropractor is a well-trained, competent primary health care provider who has undergone the scrutiny of professional and regional accreditation. The Council on Chiropractic Education in West Des Moines, Iowa, one of the two accrediting agencies that determines the curriculum and standards at chiropractic colleges, describes today's chiropractor as "a physician...who gives particular attention to the relationship of the structural and neurological aspects of the body in health and disease. [She or] he is educated in the basic and clinical sciences as well as in related health subjects. The purpose of his or her professional education is to prepare the doctor of chiropractic to be a primary health provider.... The chiropractic physician must be well trained to diagnose, including but not limited to, spinal analysis...to care for the human body in health and disease,...and to consult with, or refer to, other health care providers." [26]

The competent training and education of graduates of chiropractic colleges earns them much-deserved trust and respect in today's health care market.

Education and Training

A graduate of an accredited chiropractic college must successfully complete a five-year course of study in order to earn a degree. In order to be admitted to a chiropractic college, each student must also have at least two years of college education. Students at most chiropractic colleges are credited with more than four thousand hours of training, studying chiropractic philosophy, basic and clinical science, and clinical care in outpatient settings. Students of chiropractic learn conventional forms of medical diagnosis in addition to structural and functional diagnosis and chiropractic technique. Chiropractors also have more hours of study in neurology and radiology than most conventional medical doctors. In addition, the profession offers postgraduate training in orthopedics and radiology, and award their postgraduates with a "diplomate." Students at "straight" colleges will have as many hours but the focus of study will be narrower, i.e., "pure" chiropractic.

Licensing

Chiropractic medicine is licensed in all fifty states and the District of Columbia. In their licensing standards most states require a passing test grade from the National Board of Chiropractic Examiner's test as well as a degree from an accredited chiropractic college and two to four years of undergraduate work.

Several states also require that chiropractors pass a basic science examination similar to that required of other health practitioners. To maintain licensure, most states dictate that chiropractors complete a specific number of continuing education hours each year.

Although the scope of what is legal to practice as a chiropractic doctor varies from state to state, most chiropractors are not licensed to prescribe drugs or perform surgery, but have a broad range of other treatments and services they can provide, such as case history taking, clinical examination, laboratory tests and results, x-ray findings, evaluating emotional status, chiropractic manipulations, nutritional counseling, physical therapy, emergency procedures, exercise counseling, and disease prevention. And in some states, their license allows them to draw blood for testing and to deliver babies.

CLOSING THOUGHTS

Chiropractors can be wonderful family doctors, able to treat a wide range of illnesses and health care problems. Look for a chiropractor who will treat you and your health care needs with competency, compassion, and respect. There are many good ones in practice. Finding a chiropractor who provides the quality of care you require is worth your time and effort. Remember that approximately thirty million Americans now trust the skills and training of good chiropractic physicians for their personal health care needs. A well-trained chiropractor can be a tremendous asset to your health care team.

Chapter 10

OSTEOPATHIC MEDICINE

Structure and Function Are Two Sides of the Same Coin

Get thee knowledge of the spine for this is the requisite of understanding many diseases.

– Hippocrates

DID YOU KNOW THAT:

- Annually, 100 million patients in the United States visit osteopathic physicians.[1]

- All fifty states license osteopathic physicians to provide all types of medical services, including surgery, emergency medicine, and the prescription of drugs.[2]

- Over forty thousand osteopathic physicians are practicing in the United States.[3]

- Eighteen accredited colleges train osteopathic physicians in the United States.[4]

- On July 1, 1993, Queen Elizabeth signed the "Osteopathic's Bill," giving osteopathic medicine legal statutory recognition in Europe.[5]

- Presidents Teddy Roosevelt, Dwight D. Eisenhower, and Richard M. Nixon all used osteopathic physicians in their personal health care.[6]

- President Bill Clinton chose an osteopathic physician, Stephen Gleason, D.O., to head his panel of forty-seven medical experts to assess health care reform proposals.[7]

- Legendary athletes of the past, such as Babe Ruth, Ty Cobb, Joe DiMaggio, and golfing star Walter Hagen turned to osteopathic physicians for care. [8]
- Contemporary athletes such as Jennifer Capriati, Vitus Gerulaitus, Bjorn Borg, Lee Trevino, and members of the Chicago Bears and Washington Redskins use osteopathic physicians for their health care. [9]
- Doctors of osteopathy are team physicians to many professional athletic teams and Olympic teams. D.O.'s are also sports medical advisors to the U.S. Olympic Soccer Team, the National Soccer Team, and the Joffrey Ballet. [10]

Osteopathic physicians are on the rise. However, many consumers are confused about what they do — sometimes confusing them with chiropractors. Doctors of osteopathy (D.O.'s) are essentially M.D.'s in that they are licensed to perform all aspects of medicine, including surgery, emergency medicine, and prescribing drugs. Osteopathic physicians, however, are unique health care practitioners because they are experts in conventional medicine as well as proficient in a variety of manual treatments. These manual treatments, such as cranial manipulation, thrust technique, muscle energy, counter-strain, and myo-facial release, make changes in the musculoskeletal system that enhance the body's own healing potential. Doctors of osteopathy are also educated in a holistic perspective based on the writings of osteopathic medicine's founder, Dr. Andrew Taylor Still. As such, D.O.'s are trained to use their heads, hearts, and hands in the diagnosis and treatment of the whole patient.

The Basic Principles of Osteopathic Medicine

The principles of pure osteopathic medicine were developed by Dr. Still, a medical surgeon for the Union Army during the Civil War. Prompted by his disenchantment with the medicine of his day and the deaths of his first wife and later his three children in an epidemic of spinal meningitis, he searched for better methods to treat diseases and to promote health. During his search he developed seven principles of osteopathic medicine. These principles are:

1. A holistic perspective
2. Structure and function are interdependent
3. Blood circulation brings healing
4. The body constantly seeks balance (homeostasis)
5. The body has an inherent ability to heal itself
6. Somatic dysfunction precedes disease
7. Value and teach prevention

These seven principles taken together facilitate the goal of osteopathic medicine: a return to health.[11] In Dr. Still's own words, "To find health should be the object of the doctor. Anyone can find disease."[12] These principles may seem similar to the principles of chiropractic and naturopathic medicines; however, osteopathic physicians apply these principles in combinations unique only to osteopathic medicine. These unique combinations are achieved through the D.O.'s choice of treatments.

A holistic perspective: Since its inception, osteopathic medicine has incorporated a holistic perspective in the treatment of disease. Dr. Still believed that there were more than just physical influences that determined a person's state of health. Doctors of osteopathy who practice pure osteopathic medicine look at both the physical causes of illness as well as the role diet, exercise, emotions, attitudes, family, work, and society play. For instance, Jan Hendryx, D.O., of Boulder, Colorado tells of a case where a woman's emotional ties to her parents were the key to her recovery from chronic neck and back pain.

Dr. Hendryx's Story

When I was working in a family practice in Whitesboro, Texas, a young woman in her twenties came to see me. She stated she was suffering from chronic neck and back pain. After I examined her, I asked her if she was experiencing any stress in her life. She said that she had some stress related to her work and to her family. After she had laid down on the treatment table, I palpated [a type of examination where the physician uses his or her hands to detect tissue change such as thickening or tenderness] her neck and found the pulse or rhythm of her craniosacral system [a system of pulsing spinal and cerebral fluid which runs throughout the cranial bones and spine]. As soon as I broached the subject of this patient's parents, her cranial pulse stopped.

In osteopathic medicine, we find that there are emotional components to physical function. For instance, many times I find when I'm talking to a patient about a subject that is very sensitive to them, their cranial rhythm will completely stop. This is an example of how D.O.'s can determine important information about our patients with the use of manipulative treatments.

As this young woman and I talked more about her parents, she said her pain was increasing. I asked her to do a visualization exercise and suggested that she find within herself her "inner physician" — the power within her to help her with this pain. She did and then she shared that she felt like she had a rope tied around her neck that was choking her. I then suggested that she find a tool within herself to remove the rope. She chose some large, bright, shiny scissors and began to visualize cutting through the rope. Suddenly, she began to cry and said that the rope was her parents and that if she cut the rope, she felt her parents would die. So I then suggested that she find a more loving way to remove that rope. She directed an inner light of love on the rope to melt the rope away. Once she had done that in her mind, she told me. At that same moment, in my hands I felt a wave run through her cranial system and, immediately after, her cranial pulse returned. She began to cry and said that her neck and back pain had disappeared and that she felt a deep release and relaxation she had not felt in years. A few minutes later, she composed herself and said, "I don't really understand what just happened here, but I now know what changes I need to make in my life." [13]

Although few osteopathic physicians use imagery as a tool in their practice, classical D.O.'s use a variety of techniques founded on the principle that many illnesses have emotional, mental, and spiritual components in their cause, such as stomach ulcers, neck and back tension, skin rashes, and headaches.

Structure and function are interdependent: Just like chiropractors, doctors of osteopathic medicine consider structure (musculoskeletal system) and function (i.e., vital organ activity) to be interdependent. The D.O. works with both aspects of this essential relationship to facilitate healing. D.O.'s believe that systems of the body are interconnected. Like dominoes, when one area of the body is disrupted, reactions in other parts of the body also take place, many times leading to disease.

For example, if certain vertebrae in the back are misaligned (structure), then the organs (function) that receive their nerve impulses from that area on the spine will have some degree of dysfunction. That dysfunction can eventually lead to serious illnesses. Conversely, internal organ dysfunction can result in abnormalities in the soft tissues, muscles, and joints that can be palpated by a sensitive, knowledgeable hand. A special portion of the nervous system, called the autonomic nervous system, acts as the communication link between the outer musculoskeletal system (soma) and the internal (viscera).

Irvin M. Korr, Ph.D., during his fifty years of research in the osteopathic profession, discovered a phenomenon that validated Dr. Still's theory of this interrelationship between structure and function. This phenomenon is called, "chronic segmental facilitation." As human beings, we have a vulnerability unique from other species because we — unlike animals who have a "base" of four legs — have a close, narrow base of only two legs, as well as a vertical posture that is susceptible to gravitational shearing and torsional forces. When we receive a trauma to the spine through impact or continued inferior posture, the spinal cord becomes hypersensitized at the area of the trauma. Nerve impulses from the traumatized area are then directed to the corresponding organs and tissues located at the end of those lines of nerves. These excessive nerve pulses, over time, weaken the over-stimulated or inhibited organs or tissues on that nerve pathway, and culminate in illness. Also, a person's stress level, as well as anger, diet, and fitness level can also aggravate this hypersensitivity, contributing to a further compromise of health.

This phenomenon is one reason why classical osteopathic physicians base their practice on osteopathic manipulative therapies. According to Dr. Korr, "The primary effect of osteopathic manipulative treatment is to restore full mobility to joints by release of tensions of one or more muscles that normally move the joints by altering reflex patterns." [14]

Blood circulation brings healing: Dr. Still also emphasized the importance of stimulating blood circulation to facilitate healing. He realized that blood not only brings invaluable nutrients to cells, it also transports toxins away to the eliminative organs so they can be released from the body. Each function of circulation is essential to healing. Many times, osteopathic manual manipulations can assist the restoration of proper blood circulation where it had previously been restricted. Here's an example:

An elderly man in his seventies came to see Dr. Hendryx for a lower back pain problem. During their initial conversation, the man told Dr. Hendryx that he had arteriosclerosis, a blood circulation problem. He also shared that for years he had cold feet that always looked pale, intermittent cramping in his calves, and difficulty walking.

Dr. Hendryx palpated the man's back and found that in addition to other misaligned vertebrae, of particular note was the malalignment of his lower thoracic area. Doctors of osteopathy believe the nervous system impulses from the lower thoracic area and lower segments of the spinal cord can influence blood circulation to the lower extremities. Once Dr. Hendryx made the thoracic adjustment, the man's feet and calves immediately became pink and warm. When the man returned the next week, he reported that his feet and calves had stayed warm all week, he no longer felt cramping in his calves, and he had been able to walk better and for longer distances. [15]

Blood circulation not only brings nutrients such as vitamins and minerals to cells, but also oxygen — an essential key to health and healing.

The body constantly seeks balance (homeostasis): When the body has been injured in some way, it will attempt to adjust itself to the change in order to maintain or restore balance (homeostasis). If there is a weakened (out of balance) area that the body cannot balance, then the body attempts to balance itself around that weakened area. In essence, the body attempts to maintain balance despite the weakness. If that weakness is left untreated, it will progress from an acute, to a chronic, and finally, to a degenerative illness. One of the goals of osteopathic medicine is to help the body to balance the weakened areas so that an optimal state of homeostasis can be maintained. This increases health and vitality.

The body has an inherent ability to heal itself: Dr. Andrew Still believed that there is an innate wisdom present in the body to regulate and heal itself. Pure osteopathic medicine uses specific manipulative treatments to release and support the body's own ability to heal.

Sometimes the burden of weakened areas in the body afflicts it so much that it cannot "jump-start" its own healing powers to rejuvenate those frail or injured areas. Osteopathic treatments and regimens such as manual manipulation, physical exercise, or change of personal habits, like better nutrition, help the body to achieve a higher state of health and give the body the extra help it needs to heal.

An osteopathic physician was treating a gentleman in his sixties, who was experiencing pounding headaches. The man said, "I just don't feel right. I think my blood pressure is going up." The doctor took the man's blood pressure and it was 170/110, a full twenty points higher than the patient's usual reading. From this and other information, the physician decided to counsel the man about stress management techniques and diet. The patient agreed that he would try some breathing techniques to manage his stress but then he said, "Aren't there any treatments you can do to help me?" The D.O. told the man that there was one that might help. The doctor shares, "I did my usual cranial technique. Then, at the end, I added what is called a 'CV-4 technique.' He said, "There is an area at the brain stem that controls respiration through the autonomic nervous system. The CV-4 technique may influence that area." [16]

After the doctor made the adjustment, the gentleman took a deep breath, sighed and said that he felt much better. When the physician took the man's blood pressure again, it was 140/90 — a substantial drop in ten minutes.

When the man came back the following week, he reported that the pounding in his head had disappeared and that his blood pressure had been fine all week.

Somatic dysfunction precedes disease: Osteopathic physicians believe that the body comes into a state of "holding" or "restriction" before it actually becomes ill or diseased. D.O.'s seek to identify those areas that are in "somatic dysfunction" and use the appropriate treatments to heal those areas before they degenerate into an illness.

Value and teach prevention: Like most alternative practitioners, osteopathic physicians believe an important part of their job is to educate their patients in the prevention of disease. In order to do this, they receive part of their formal education in nutrition, exercise, and healthy lifestyle choices. In fact, osteopathic medicine places such an emphasis on prevention that it offers a specialty in preventative medicine.

Dr. Hendryx had a personal experience with the value of preventative medicine — specifically through exercise. He says, "At the Texas College of Osteopathic Medicine, we were required to take a class entitled 'Personal Wellness.' Among the topics covered in this class was exercise physiology and how it affects health. As part of our requirements for passing this class, we had to design an exercise program for ourselves. At the time, I was in my late twenties and had significant lower back pain that was so severe that some days it was difficult for me to get out of bed. I had this condition for quite a while. Through the fitness program that I designed for myself in this class, I began to strengthen my back with exercise and stretching. Before long, my back pain had gone. And today, as long as I keep my back strong, it continues to be pain free.

"I share this story with many of my patients who need some extra prodding toward exercise. I explain to them that since we are usually sedentary during our days, it is easy for the body to lose its strength. Physical strength is not just for lifting heavy objects or to throw a baseball a far distance, we also need it to structurally hold our bodies in an optimal posture. One of my most favorite quotes is from Dr. Viola Frymann. She said, 'Life is motion and motion is life.'" [17]

Osteopathic physicians have long been noted for their commitment to teach their patients how to avoid illness and how to maintain and enhance their health. For this reason, many athletes of the past and present seek the advice of osteopathic physicians to heighten their performance, and to prevent injury and illness.

Osteopathic Physicians: A Difference in Treatment Philosophy

Since its inception, the evolution of osteopathic medicine has been influenced by the presence and power of conventional medicine. One result of this influence is that three distinct groups of osteopathic physicians exist today.

Harold Magoun, Jr., D.O., F.A.A.O., a fellow of the American Academy of Osteopathy and a respected elder of the profession, says, "There is a minority of us who practice "pure" osteopathy, another minority who practice pure [conventional] medicine, and a large group of D.O.'s who use some manipulation along with their medical, surgical, and obstetrical practice." [18]

The first group are the D.O.'s who practice osteopathy founded on the principles and techniques developed by Dr. Still and other early pioneers of osteopathic medicine. These D.O.'s use manipulative techniques as their primary way of implementing the osteopathic principles. It is estimated that only 5 to 10 percent of all osteopathic physicians in practice are in this group.

The second group of D.O.'s, who are also a minority, practice conventional medicine and do not use manipulative treatments on their patients. For the most part, in practice, they are very similar to a conventional medical doctor (M.D.), and therefore, do not usually adhere to the seven principles of osteopathy as discussed earlier in this chapter.

The third group, by far the largest group, practice a combination of conventional medicine and manipulative treatments. D.O.'s in this group adhere to osteopathic principles in varying degrees in the practice of their medicine.

This difference can mean a completely different style of care from one osteopathic physician to another. This disparity of treatment priorities is rooted in osteopathic medicine's historical fight for legitimacy.

Initially osteopathic medicine and allopathic or conventional medicine traded negative but harmless criticisms. The AMA called osteopathic physicians "cultists" while Dr. Still called conventional doctors "poisoners." [19]

However, as the AMA gained economic and political power, its ambition to eliminate or assimilate competitive systems of medicine also grew. In the late 1930s, Dr. Charles Spencer, a renowned osteopathic physician of his day, and a student of Dr. Still, stated his serious concern that the allopathic medical profession would use its political power to absorb osteopathy. He feared that if that assimilation occurred, the unique treatments and philosophies of osteopathic medicine would be lost forever. [20]

Then, in California in 1962, the AMA attempted to do just that.

Its political machinery put a bill in motion that banned osteopathic medicine in California. The twelve hundred osteopathic
physicians in California were given a choice to buy an M.D.
license for $65 or to stop practicing in California altogether.
Approximately three-fourths of practicing D.O.'s at the time
chose the M.D. degree. In fact, the college that Dr. Charles
Spencer had helped establish decades before, The Los Angeles
College of Osteopathic Medicine, was absorbed into the conventional medicine school system. [21]

In 1974 the ban against osteopathic physicians practicing in
California was overturned by the courts. However, as a result of
the California experience, the osteopathic profession realized
that its very survival was at stake. In an attempt to survive the
scrutiny and bias of the powerful conventional medical community, the profession as a whole made a decision to identify itself
as "mainstream medicine," having equal standing with M.D.'s in
the community. [22]

Many within the profession feel that in their attempt to protect their professional reputation in this way, D.O.'s have allowed
conventional medicine to influence them too much. Dr. Magoun
says, "Many osteopathic physicians have tried so hard to be as
good as M.D.'s that they have become M.D.'s." [23]

As a result of this, much of the healing wisdom and many of
the principles that were the foundation of osteopathic medicine
have been compromised. Today it is estimated that approximately one out of every three practicing D.O.'s does not use
osteopathic manipulation in his or her practice. [24]

The *American Holistic Health Association Complete Guide to Alternative Medicine* says, "The majority [of osteopathic physicians] liber-
ally use allopathic approaches in their practice and align
themselves politically and professionally with allopathy,
although some augment their practice with osteopathic manipulation. To many of these, osteopathic medical education was
mainly a vehicle for becoming a licensed physician and the
unique heritage of the tradition is not emphasized so much in
their practice." [25]

The 5 to 10 percent who use manipulative therapies as the foundation of their practice have been described as the "torch bearers" of the pure principles of osteopathic medicine. Most of these D.O.'s belong to the American Academy of Osteopathy (AAO). AAO's membership is approximately two thousand osteopathic physicians, as compared to the almost forty thousand D.O.'s practicing in the United States.

Despite the small numbers of D.O.'s practicing pure osteopathic medicine, Dr. Magoun is optimistic that the numbers of osteopathic physicians using manipulative therapies will continue to rise in the future. "The students we are graduating today are well trained and excited about manipulative techniques," he says. "The teachers are instilling enthusiasm about the possibilities that these treatments hold for them as practicing physicians." [26] However, in today's medical market, consumers who want to work with D.O.'s who specialize in manipulative therapies still need to actively seek them out.

DISTINCTIONS BETWEEN CHIROPRACTORS AND OSTEOPATHIC PHYSICIANS

Both chiropractors (D.C.'s) and osteopathic physicians (D.O.'s) offer a range of manipulative treatments. However, there are some important differences between them, namely education and licensure.

Chiropractors are well versed in the clinical and basic sciences, as are osteopathic physicians. However, the clinical education obtained through hospital-based residencies of the D.O. provide an in-depth knowledge of illness and disease that goes beyond that of chiropractors. For this reason, D.O.'s are trained to perform a more thorough diagnostic exam. D.O.'s are also licensed to prescribe drugs in all states as well as to perform surgery, whereas chiropractors cannot.

Still, if you are seeking manipulative treatments for your health care needs, chiropractors merit consideration. This is especially true if the osteopathic physicians available to you do not offer manipulative therapies as a primary form of treatment. In such cases, a chiropractor would be a better choice if you want to be competently treated with manipulative techniques.

The Four Major Treatments of Classical Osteopathic Medicine

The four major treatments of osteopathic medicine include manipulation, nutrition and diet, exercise, and pharmaceutical drugs.

Osteopathic Manipulations

Osteopathic medicine provides many methods of manual manipulation designed to improve posture and musculoskeletal function and, therefore, to support the body's innate healing processes. The importance of using manipulation to enhance healing is increasingly being noted by health care professionals of various systems of medicine. Andrew Weil, M.D., says in his book *Health and Healing*, "Manipulation seems to me a good technique to know. I wish I had learned it in medical school. It can be a valuable addition to a doctor's therapeutic repertory, both because it involves a laying on of hands that can foster productive relationships with patients, and because it may improve the circulation of blood and nervous energy to ailing parts of the body. Furthermore, the importance of the skeletal system is underrated by allopaths, and even by orthopedists, who are supposed to be scientific experts on bones." [27] The importance of the skeletal system in healing is a core premise in osteopathy.

Leon Chaitow, N.D., D.O., is both an osteopathic physician and a naturopathic physician. He says, "The musculoskeletal system makes up the largest body system, using far and away the greatest amount of energy. If you reflect on the fact that it is through this musculoskeletal system that you live your life, you will begin to appreciate osteopathy's importance." [28]

Manipulative techniques are quite clearly the cornerstone of classical osteopathy. They can range from subtle, gentle pressure that move bodily fluids such as blood, lymph, and cerebrospinal fluid, to more active manipulations that move solid components of the musculoskeletal structure like fascia, muscles, bones, tendons, and ligaments. The following are some examples of those methods:

Thrust Technique is perhaps the most widely recognized form of manual manipulation. With this technique the D.O. uses a "high velocity-low amplitude" movement. This movement can be applied to the spine and the extremities to restore normal position and function. Once a joint returns to its optimal position, tenderness and restriction of motion quickly disappear.

Our three-year-old son, John, went to see an osteopathic physician when he complained that his neck hurt. After one application of the thrust technique, we asked him if his neck still hurt. His response was, "Not any more!"

Cranial Techniques — Cranial manipulation or cranial osteopathy was developed by William Sutherland, D.O., in the 1930s when he observed that cranial bones are mobile and can be gently moved with the hands. Sutherland went on to theorize that when cranial bones are not free to move, it adversely affects the twelve cranial nerves, the pituitary gland, the vital centers in the brain stem, and the whole body. When cranial nerve function is compromised, it can affect the vital functioning of vision, digestion, or respiration, thus making one more susceptible to illness. Restoring freedom of motion of the cranial bones can help to restore those vital functions as well as some aspects of endocrine and cerebral function.

Today in La Jolla, California, Viola Frymann, D.O., specializes in cranial osteopathy and has found it tremendously helpful for children who have sustained head injuries at birth. On Oct. 3, 1990, a reporter for the *Los Angeles Times* described one of Dr. Frymann's sessions with a two-year-old girl:

"The little girl lay on the examination table, crying so violently that her body arched upward. Her eyes rolled wildly and her tongue jutted stiffly out of her mouth. The keening sound vibrated off the wall and seemed to stun everyone in the tiny room to numb silence.

"Everyone but the doctor. Crooning, 'All is well, all is well,' Dr. Viola Frymann approached the two-year-old. Frymann rolled the small girl over and slowly rubbed her back. Next, she cupped her hand around the child's head and gently pressed. Behind her, a woman played a Beethoven sonata on the piano.

"After what seemed like forever, but was only ten minutes, the child's cry slowed to a small moan. Frymann then moved a small, colorful toy in front of the little girl's eyes and the child tracked it.

"'That's wonderful!' Frymann said to her. 'You know, you've never been interested in things like this before!' It was the first time the little girl had ever paid any attention to toys."[29] In only ten minutes, Dr. Frymann had created a dramatic change in this child's life.

Recently, Dr. Frymann opened the "Osteopathic Center for Children," devoted to treating birth-injured children, and training osteopathic physicians in this special art. [30]

In addition to facilitating spectacular progress in brain-damaged children, cranial osteopathy also helps more common ailments, such as headaches and migraines. It may also help heal such diverse maladies as hypoglycemia, pneumonia, and heart disease.

Muscle Energy technique is a widely used approach where restrictions of motion are diagnosed, and under the physician's direction, the patient then uses his or her own muscle power to restore normal function. This was developed by Fred Mitchel, Sr., D.O.

Myofascial Release is a technique to loosen "fixed" connective tissue that surrounds muscles. When the connective tissue becomes fixed through injury or trauma, it is almost impossible for the area to relax or "release." With deep manual manipulation of both the muscles and fascia (connective tissue), the area loosens, becoming relaxed.

Counter-strain was developed by Larry Jones, D.O., in which the patient is placed in the position the strain occurred, the tissues are allowed to relax, and then the patient is slowly returned to a neutral position.

Soft-Tissue Techniques are usually applied on the muscles around the spine. It entails stretching, deep pressure, and traction. The goal is to relax the muscles, and to move fluids or decrease edema, thus reestablishing removal of toxins and reestablishing circulation. This brings movement and renewed vitality in areas of somatic dysfunction.

Visceral Manipulation technique is used by D.O.'s to treat internal organs by applying gentle pressure through the abdominal wall. This technique facilitates correct positioning of the organ, improves its circulation and lymphatic drainage, and helps the organ move in its normal range of motion, thus improving function. A thirty-five-year-old woman went to see her osteopathic physician after seeing her family M.D. She had been experiencing a "burning" sensation in her stomach. Her M.D. had prescribed Tagamet after he concluded that she had an ulcer. She told her D.O. that the Tagamet had helped but that her stomach still bothered her. Her D.O. asked her if her mid-back was at all uncomfortable. She responded that it was *very* uncomfortable. The D.O. was not surprised that her mid-back was tight since it is considered a reflex area to the stomach. The muscles and the stomach had become *reflexively* linked through the spinal chord in a vicious cycle.

The D.O. did some osteopathic manipulation to her back, and then did a visceral manipulation on her stomach to loosen some of the "tightness" of the organ. The next week the woman reported that both her back and her stomach were much better and that she had cut down the amount of Tagamet "quite a bit."

Other manual manipulative techniques used by D.O.'s include lymphatic pump, joint mobilization, strain-counterstrain, and other positioning techniques.

Nutrition and Diet

Nutritional recommendations of osteopathic physicians mirror the accepted dietary and nutritional standards of today. This includes low-fat, high-fiber foods and vitamin and mineral support.

In addition, D.O.'s use nutrition for preventative medicine. For instance, to prevent coronary heart disease, many D.O.'s recommend their patients avoid fats, especially saturated fats. Dr. Hendryx suggests that his patients take 1,000 – 4,000 mg of Vitamin C, 8,000 i.u. of Vitamin A, and 1,000 i.u. of Vitamin E daily. He says that these antioxidants help prevent free radical formation, thus preventing tissue breakdown as well as the accumulation of plaque in the arteries.

Exercise

Exercise has always been an important treatment of osteopathic medicine because the physical exertion of exercise supports the concept that structure and function are interdependent and interrelated. When patients exercise, they strengthen their muscular structure. By doing this, they are also supporting the healthy function of their vital organs.

Osteopathic physicians also see that health is compromised by a *lack* of exercise. Essentially, a life without exercise results in the eventual dysfunction of vital organs. Dr. Charles Spencer was an athlete in his younger years and studied the cause and treatment of injuries to athletes during his over thirty-five years of practice. As a result, athletes of legendary status such as Babe Ruth and Joe DiMaggio sought his expertise. In 1925 he wrote, "Exercise is the most fundamental of biologic laws. Nature harbors no drones. Cells that stop work begin to lose their capacity to function, and if not exercised they ultimately die." [31]

This focus on exercise makes osteopathic medicine a logical choice for care among athletes. As such, many D.O.'s actively practice sports medicine for the amateur as well the professional athlete.

Pharmaceutical Drugs

Andrew Still did not believe in the use of pharmaceutical drugs. He believed that the innate healing ability of the human body was sufficient to heal illnesses and diseases. However, even Dr. Still's first graduates of osteopathic medicine used drugs as an adjunct to manipulative therapies. Today's classical or pure osteopathic physician prescribes pharmaceuticals when medically necessary, such as antibiotics for pneumonia or pain relievers for chronic pain.

Dr. Spencer's Story: My Introduction to Osteopathic Medicine

I had painful migraines in my early years and tried various methods and remedies to cure them. Despite my efforts, several times a year the pain was so severe that I was forced to bed. I certainly didn't enjoy these headaches, but I feel that they were somewhat of a blessing to me because they inspired me to want to help other people in pain. Consequently, I had planned to be a doctor of allopathy [conventional medicine].

One day I was traveling in Missouri and I came upon a public exhibition. As I walked closer, I saw that it was a demonstration of a new medicine called osteopathy by a Dr. Andrew Still. Since I had an interest in medicine, I stayed to hear him talk.

Dr. Still called out to the crowd a list of illnesses and maladies that he was convinced osteopathy could cure. He requested volunteers from the audience who might have these illnesses so that he could show the crowd osteopathy's great value. One of the illnesses he mentioned was migraines, and since I felt one coming on that morning, I quickly volunteered.

When I stepped up onto the platform, Dr. Still had me lie on a long makeshift table. Once on my back, he felt my spine and my neck with his fingers, then he bent my back in such a manner that a series of "pops" occurred, which for a moment concerned me. Next, he gently twisted my neck and again I heard a slight "pop." Any concern I had at the time quickly left when I realized that my migraine had disappeared.

After the demonstration, I went to Dr. Still and respectfully insisted that he show me exactly how he had cured me of the migraine. He was quite agreeable. He called it "lightning bone setting." First he showed me which vertebrae in my neck and back he found malaligned, then how he moved them.

Once I understood the technique, I boarded the nearest train and hurried back home to Normal, Ohio, to see my sister. She had suffered the same migraines as I. Once I arrived, I told her about Dr. Still and how he had helped my migraine. I suggested that she allow me to try the technique on her, and she was glad to have me try. When I applied the technique on her neck and back, her migraine also disappeared.

These events convinced me that osteopathy was a medicine I wanted to study. In 1902, I graduated from the S.S. Still School of Osteopathy and was eager to help people with the powerful knowledge I now had. [32]

HEALTH CONDITIONS THAT RESPOND WELL TO OSTEOPATHIC MEDICINE

Osteopathic medicine is best known for healing conditions of the musculoskeletal system such as headaches, neck and back pain, or injuries that have occurred during car accidents or sports activities. Besides the millions of testimonials from satisfied patients over the last one hundred years, osteopathic medicine also has a large body of scientific research to document its efficacy. [33]

For example, one such study validated osteopathic medicine's ability to help lower back pain. The study focused on the results of osteopathic manipulation on the lumbar vertebrae of twenty-six people. The participating D.O.'s used the thrust technique to accomplish the adjustments. Researchers found that this technique decreased muscle tension during movement and lessened muscle spasm and lower back pain. [34]

Osteopathic physicians contend that their medicine can help heal such illnesses as asthma, bronchitis, pneumonia, stomach problems, hypertension, anginal pain, menstrual pain, and ear infections. Classical D.O.'s help heal these various illnesses by stimulating the healing properties of the body by manipulative techniques. [35]

One particular study entitled, "The efficacy of OMT in the elderly hospitalized with acute pneumonia," focused on aged patients. These patients were receiving antibiotics for pneumonia while they were hospitalized. The researchers found that the patients who received manual manipulation as part of their treatment regimen required fewer antibiotics and were able to leave the hospital sooner than those patients who did not receive manipulative therapy. [36]

Viola Frymann, D.O., has helped many young patients suffering from ear infections by treating them with osteopathic treatments. "We get children with recurrent ear infections that started when they were six months old and have gone on for years," she says. "Parents are sick of the merry-go-round of antibiotics and ear infections. When we begin to address the structural problem, which may have originated at birth, the ear infections become progressively less frequent." [37]

Osteopathic medicine can also be helpful for patients with heart conditions. In some cases of heart dysfunction, the cause of the problem is not the heart itself but the skeletal structure surrounding the heart, which affects the nerve supply to the heart. Dr. Harold Magoun recounts a story detailing how the renowned D.L. Clark, an osteopathic pioneer in Texas and Colorado, relieved a man from heart distress and saved his life:

"In the early 1870s, Dr. Clark was called to see the president of a major railroad company in Denver, Colorado. The man had such a high heart rate that his physicians couldn't count them.

They had given the patient various drugs to slow his heart, but none of them had much effect on the patient's dangerously high heart rate. Therefore, the M.D.'s told the man's family that the man had a matter of hours to live.

"His family asked the physicians if they could call Dr. Clark as a last resort. The physicians agreed, saying that since the man was about to die, there wasn't anything Dr. Clark could do to harm him. Dr. Clark arrived and took the history of the patient, then examined him. After finding a malalignment in the upper back, he used osteopathic manipulations to treat him. After Dr. Clark had completed his manipulations, the man threw up his hands and sighed. The M.D.'s said, 'Oh, my God. He's killed him!' But the patient said, 'No, that's the first moment of relief I've had!' Soon after, the patient's heart rate slowed to a normal rate and this president of the railroad company was an osteopathic convert." During his life, Dr. Clark treated legislators and was a significant force in establishing osteopathic licensure in Texas and Colorado. [38]

Osteopathic medicine has been a favorite of athletes almost since its inception because D.O.'s offer effective solutions to healing an injury that do not involve surgery. In addition, athletes may receive valuable information about why the injury happened in the first place. Mitchel Story, D.O., medical director of the Sports Medicine Clinic in Seattle says, "There's a difference in the way a runner would be evaluated by a D.O. versus an M.D. We may pick up some flaws in the mechanics of the pelvis, and from a gait analysis and treadmill evaluation we might detect minor deviations in the ranges of motion of the hips and knees." [39] Information such as this can prevent further injuries as well as enhance sports performance.

Osteopathic medicine has had a colorful history of quickly healing serious health problems. Some patients with minor health problems, however, find that symptoms that seemed unrelated to their original complaint have also been helped. Anthony D. Capobianco, D.O., says, "A lot of people associate [osteopathy] with problems like lower back pain, and that's okay because during a treatment other parts of their body respond. The next time a patient comes in, they'll say, 'By the way, my hay fever is better.' They begin to understand that osteopathy is available to them for virtually anything."[40] Experiences like these also help patients understand the healing relationship between structure and function.

Applying the Five Steps to Osteopathic Medicine

When you have decided to use the skills and services of an osteopathic physician, it is in your best interest to find out as much as you can about who the physician is and how he or she will treat you before you agree to treatment. Here are some suggestions to help you identify whether a particular doctor of osteopathic medicine will be the right caregiver for you.

Additions to Step Two: Get Good Referrals

All osteopathic physicians are well trained in conventional medicine as well as in the basic principles of osteopathic medicine. This extensive education by itself makes any osteopathic physician a unique and valuable health care provider. However, it is that special 5 to 10 percent of all D.O.'s who practice classical or pure osteopathy, using manipulative therapies as the foundation of their practice who seem most valuable as practitioners of "alternative medicine."

If you desire treatment from a classical osteopathic physician, your best bet is to contact the American Academy of Osteopathy (AAO). For $5 they will send you a list of their members who practice in your state. Their approximately two thousand members use manipulative therapies as a primary treatment in their practice.

The largest association for osteopathic physicians is the American Osteopathic Association (AOA). They are considered the principal association for this profession. If you contact the AOA, they will provide you with a list of their D.O. members practicing in your area. Remember that D.O. members of this association may or may not use manipulative therapies.

Additions to Step Three: Screen the Candidate

Asking well-targeted questions to the staff of an osteopathic physician gives you valuable information about the caregiver before you make your first appointment. Add the following questions to Step Three: Screen the Candidates. Using all the questions will give you a good first glance at this professional and valuable information to help you decide whether this is the D.O. you'll want to work with.

Here are questions we suggest asking the staff or your potential osteopathic physician directly:

Can I expect the doctor to use manipulative therapies during my treatment?

Approximately one-third of all D.O.'s choose not to use their manipulative training in their practice. If manipulative therapies are important to you, make sure this D.O. will provide them during your treatment.

How long are sessions with the doctor?

D.O.'s who practice like conventional M.D.'s consult for only twelve to fifteen minutes during an appointment. A D.O. who practices pure osteopathic medicine will take much more time than that. A classical D.O. will spend time taking an extensive history, as well as performing one or more osteopathic manipulative techniques.

What training has the doctor had in treatments not taught in osteopathic medical school?

Although graduates of osteopathic medical colleges are trained in some alternative-care treatments, they are not trained in all of them.

If this D.O. practices homeopathy, acupuncture, or any other alternative treatment outside his or her original medical college training, ask how many hours of training this doctor has, and if he or she earned any certifications or degrees from this training. The answers to these questions will help you determine if this D.O. is competently trained in the alternative treatments they offer.

WHAT TO EXPECT DURING AN APPOINTMENT WITH A CLASSICAL OSTEOPATHIC PHYSICIAN

The initial visit with an osteopathic physician specializing in pure osteopathic techniques and theories is in some ways just like an initial meeting with an M.D. The D.O. will take a health history as well as hear details about a patient's physical complaint. The usual tests will be administered — blood pressure, heart and respiration rates — as well as other conventional medical tests like x-rays or blood tests if necessary.

From that point, the session will be distinctly different from a session with an M.D. The classical D.O. will ask the patient to lie on a padded treatment table where the D.O. will gently palpate or touch the patient's body to lead the physician to more detail about the patient's problem. This palpation includes feeling and pressing areas of the body that are painful or tense. D.O.'s trained in the classical arts of osteopathy use their hands to help discover tenderness, swelling, stiffness, or thickening of soft tissues and accompanying dysfunctions in joints or the cranium. Palpation assists the doctor in assessing the root cause of the patient's complaint.

The doctor then chooses one or more manipulative therapies to help the patient's particular problem. If the doctor chooses cranial manipulation, the doctor will make subtle and sometimes barely perceptible movements. On the other hand, if the doctor chooses a thrust technique, the physician will use enough force to make the correct adjustment, usually to the spine. Most manipulative treatment sessions are pain free and sessions can last a half hour or longer.

Once the physician has finished the manipulations, he or she may suggest exercises or dietary changes for the patient. Or the physician may decide to use another therapy such as acupuncture or homeopathy to further support the patient's healing.

Before the first session is finished, the doctor should discuss how much time and how many treatments are required to heal the patient's health problem. For an acute problem, as little as one to two treatments may be all that is required to correct it. The number and frequency of treatment is tailored to the patient's ability to heal and usually does not exceed two treatments per week. For more chronic conditions, usually twelve to sixteen treatments may be prescribed over a three-month period. Serious conditions may warrant six months or more of osteopathic treatments. The osteopathic physician will attempt to do as much as the body can accept each time to minimize the number of treatments.

COST AND INSURANCE

Cost

The fees for using osteopathic physicians may be less than those of conventional medical doctors if the D.O. utilizes mostly manipulative treatments. Also, if a health condition warrants drugs and high-tech medical procedures, the cost is about the same as that of an M.D. "Because of their palpatory skills," Dr. Magoun states, "osteopathic physicians can frequently arrive at a correct diagnosis without unnecessary lab tests, x-rays, scans, and MRIs." [41]

Insurance

Given that D.O.'s are licensed to provide the same services as M.D.'s, the coverage and reimbursement are similar to that of conventional medical doctors.

EDUCATION, TRAINING, AND LICENSING

Education and Training

As earlier stated, osteopathic physicians are trained exactly as conventional doctors except that D.O.'s have additional training related to osteopathic principles and procedures. For example, they have more training in preventative medicine such as nutrition, diet, and exercise. In addition, they are trained in manual manipulative techniques. Osteopathic physicians graduate from a four-year medical school, complete a residency program, pass comparable state boards, and practice in fully accredited and licensed hospitals.

Unlike chiropractors, who are also licensed to perform manipulative therapies, D.O.'s are trained to prescribe drugs, to diagnose and treat all pathologies (illness and diseases), and to perform surgery and emergency medicine. Dr. Capobianco says, "Even before the first osteopathic treatment is performed, the doctor has handled cardiac codes, delivered babies, and has assisted in major surgery. Unless you study medicine and surgery, there will be important and dangerous limitations." [42]

Like conventional medical doctors, doctors of osteopathic medicine earn specialties in different modalities of medicine — forty-eight of them, such as pediatrics, family medicine, internal medicine, obstetrics, gynecology, and psychiatry. Many classical osteopathic physicians have earned a certification of specialty in osteopathic manipulative medicine from the American Academy of Osteopathy.

Licensing

In most states, osteopathic physicians, like M.D.'s, are permitted under the scope of their licenses to do any treatment that is safe and necessary for their patient's health. There are exceptions to this. For example, they must pass special exams to practice acupuncture in New Mexico and homeopathy in Arizona. Also, in some states a minimum number of hours of study are required to practice acupuncture, ranging from two hundred to one thousand hours.

CLOSING THOUGHTS

With such vast technical training in preventative medicine, manipulative therapies, conventional medicine, and the holistic perspective, osteopathic medicine makes the D.O. one of the most versatile and well-trained providers of alternative medicine. Andrew Weil, M.D., in his book *Spontaneous Healing*, described the doctor of the future as having a combination of conventional medical expertise, alternative medical skills, and a holistic perspective. Clearly the doctor of the future is here today: the pure or classical osteopathic physician. ▪

REFERENCES

HOW TO MAKE ALTERNATIVE MEDICINE WORK FOR YOU

1. NIH. *Alternative Medicine: Expanding Medical Horizons* (U.S. Government Printing Office, 1993), 183.

2. "Mapping Medicines Movements," *Vegetarian Times*, October 1994, 78; William Collinge. *The American Holistic Health Association Complete Guide to Alternative Medicine* (Warner Books, 1996), 42–43.

3. Mark Kastner and Hugh Burroughs. *Alternative Healing: The Complete A to Z Guide to Over 160 Alternative Therapies* (Halcyon Publishing, 1993), 3.

4. Bill Gottlieb. *New Choices in Natural Healing* (Rodale Press, Inc., 1995), 4.

5. *Complementary and Alternative Medicine at the* NIH, Volume III, Number 1, 3.

6. *American Demographics*, July 1993, 16.

7. *Complementary and Alternative Medicine at the* NIH, Volume III, Number 1, 1.

8. Burton Goldberg. *Alternative Medicine: The Definitive Guide* (Future Medicine Publishing, 1993), 15.

9. Norman Cousins. Personal interview, January 1990.

10. James F. Fries, M.D. and Donald M. Vickery, M.D. *Take Care of Yourself* (Addison-Wesley Co., 1989), 116.

11. Adriane Fugh-Berman, M.D. "The Case for 'Natural' Medicine," *The Nation*, September 6/13, 1993, 242.

12. Burton Goldberg. *Alternative Medicine: The Definitive Guide* (Future Medicine Publishing, 1993), 5.

13. Bill Gottlieb. *New Choices in Natural Healing* (Rodale Press, Inc., 1995), 3.

14. NIH. *Alternative Medicine: Expanding Medical Horizons* (U.S. Government Printing Office, 1993), liv.

15. Ibid, xiv.

16. Ibid, xiv.

17. Ibid, xv.

18. Ibid, 2.

19. AMA Resolution #514, "Alternative (Complementary) Medicine," Reference Committee E, 10–11.

20. Fact Sheet #1, "Alternative Medical Courses Taught at U.S. Medical Schools," The Richard and Hinda Rosenthal Center for Alternative/Complementary Medicine.

21. "Unconventional Claims," *Vegetarian Times*, October 1995, 27.

22. Deirdre O'Conner, N.D. The Naturopathic Model of Primary Care Natural Medicine. Presentation at "Integrating Managed Care & Alternative Medicine," San Francisco, CA, December 1, 1995.

23. David Eisenberg, M.D. "Unconventional Medicine in the United States," *New England Journal of Medicine*, January 28, 1993, 246.

24. Burton Goldberg. *Alternative Medicine: The Definitive Guide* (Future Medicine Publishing, 1993), 450.

25. William Collinge. *The American Holistic Health Association Complete Guide to Alternative Medicine* (Warner Books, 1996), 40.

26. Martha Ullman at the National Center for Homeopathy. Personal communication, July, 1996.

27. Donald J. Brown, N.D. The Use of Herbal Medicine in a Clinical Setting. Presentation at "Integrating Managed Care & Alternative Medicine," San Francisco, CA, December 1995.

28. B. Hayes. U.S. "Survey of Insurers." Government study, HEW as reported by The American Chiropractic Association, Arlington,

VA, November 1995.

29. Bill Gottlieb. *New Choices in Natural Healing* (Rodale Press, Inc, 1995), 3.

30. David Eisenberg, M.D. "Unconventional Medicine in the United States," *New England Journal of Medicine*, January 28, 1993, 246.

31. Ibid.

32. Ibid.

33. Ibid.

34. John Weeks. "Charting the Mainstream: A Review of Trends in the Dominant Medical System," *Townsend Letter*, Port Townsend, Washington, February/March 1996, 38–39.

35. Len Wisneski, M.D. Personal interview, September 1989.

36. Joe Jacobs, M.D. Personal interview, November 1995.

37. NIH. *Alternative Medicine: Expanding Medical Horizons* (U.S. Government Printing Office, 1993), xiii.

38. Andrew L. Shapiro. *We're Number One* (Vintage Books, 1992), 4, 16, 22, 25, 27, 28.

39. Bill Gottlieb. *New Choices in Natural Healing* (Rodale Press, Inc, 1995), 7.

40. Hassan S. Rafaat, M.D. Integrating Alternative Medicine into the Mainstream: the Answer to an Ailing Health Care System. Presentation at "Integrating Managed Care & Alternative Medicine," San Francisco, CA, December 1995.

41. Washington State, House Bill 1046, 1995.

CHAPTER ONE: LEARN YOUR OPTIONS

1. Norman Cousins. Personal interview, January 1990.

2. Carol Ann Barry. "Taking Charge of your Health," *Family Circle*, April 25, 1995, 35.

3. Christiane Northrup, M.D. Personal interview, September 1989.

4. Joan Borysenko, Ph.D. "The Best Medicine," *New Age Journal*,

May/June 1990, 43.

5. Mary Walker. "Surviving AIDS," *East/West Journal*, January 1991, 39.

6. World Research Foundation brochure.

7. Hermes Consumer Medical Search Service brochure.

8. Lloyd J. Ney. Personal interview, March 1996.

9. Joan Borysenko, Ph.D. "The Best Medicine," *New Age Journal*, May/June 1991, 39.

CHAPTER TWO: GET GOOD REFERRALS

1. Bernie Siegel, M.D. Personal interview, November 1989.

2. Alan Adams, M.D. Personal interview, September 1989.

CHAPTER THREE: SCREEN THE CANDIDATES

1. Lawrence C. Horowitz, M.D. *Taking Charge of Your Medical Fate* (Random House, 1988), xv.

2. Christiane Northrup, M.D. Personal interview, September 1989.

3. John E. Upledger, D.O. Personal interview, September 1989.

4. Bernie Siegel, M.D. Personal interview, November 1989.

CHAPTER FOUR: INTERVIEW THE PROVIDER

1. Larry Dossey, M.D. Personal interview, December 1989.

2. Leonard Wisneski, M.D. Personal interview, September 1989.

3. Larry Dossey, M.D. Personal interview, December 1989.

4. Ibid.

5. Christiane Northrup, M.D. Personal interview, December 1989.

6. Larry Dossey, M.D. Personal interview, September 1989.

7. Ibid.

8. Joan Borysenko, Ph.D. "The Best Medicine," *New Age Journal*, May/June 1991, 39.

9. Ibid.

CHAPTER FIVE: FORM A PARTNERSHIP

1. David Hibbard, M.D. Personal interview, September 1989.

2. Norman Cousins. Personal interview, January 1990.

3. Len Wisneski, M.D. Personal interview, September 1989.

4. Stanley Krippner, Ph.D. Personal interview, October 1989.

5. David R. Stutz, M.D. and Bernard Feder, Ph.D. *The Savvy Patient* (Consumer Reports Books,1990), 78.

6. John Upledger, D.O. Personal interview, Fall 1989

7. Larry Dossey, M.D. Personal interview, December 1989.

8. Christiane Northrup, M.D. Personal interview, September 1989.

9. Bernie Siegel, M.D. Personal interview, August 1989.

10. David R. Stutz, M.D. and Bernard Feder, Ph.D. *The Savvy Patient* (Consumer Reports Books, 1990), 87.

11. Michael Toms. "Roots of Healing: The New Medicine," *Alternative Therapies*, May 1995, 46.

12. Joan Borysenko, Ph.D. "The Best Medicine," *New Age Journal*, May/June 1991, 39.

13. Mary Walker. "Surviving AIDS," *East/West Journal*, January 1991, 39.

THE TERRAIN OF ALTERNATIVE MEDICINE

1. Television advertisement for health care books.

2. Brad M. Hayes, D.C. Strategies for Integrating Chiropractic into Managed Care Setting. Presentation at "Integrating Managed Care & Alternative Medicine," San Francisco, CA, December 1995.

3. NIH. *Alternative Medicine: Expanding Medical Horizons* (U.S. Government Printing Office, 1993), 76.

4. Ibid, 183.

5. Donald J. Brown, N.D. The Use of Herbal Medicine in a Clinical Setting. Presentation at "Integrating Managed Care & Alternative Medicine," San Francisco, CA, December 1995.

6. Burton Goldberg. *Alternative Medicine: The Definitive Guide* (Future Medicine Publishing, 1993), 37–45; William Collinge. *The American Holistic Health Association Complete Guide to Alternative Medicine* (Warner Books, 1996), 13–47; NIH. *Alternative Medicine: Expanding Medical Horizons* (U.S. Government Printing Office, 1993), 5–79.

7. Mark Kastner and Hugh Burroughs. *Alternative Healing: The Complete A to Z Guide to Over 160 Alternative Therapies* (Halcyon Publishing, 1993), 2.

8. Ibid, 20.

9. Burton Goldberg. *Alternative Medicine: The Definitive Guide* (Future Medicine Publishing, 1993), 73–79.

10. Ibid, 127–133.

11. Mark Kastner and Hugh Burroughs. *Alternative Healing: The Complete A to Z Guide to Over 160 Alternative Therapies* (Halcyon Publishing, 1993), 59–62.

12. Ibid, 62–64.

13. Burton Goldberg. *Alternative Medicine: The Definitive Guide* (Future Medicine Publishing, 1993), 319–329.

14. Mark Kastner and Hugh Burroughs. *Alternative Healing: The Complete A to Z Guide to Over 160 Alternative Therapies* (Halcyon Publishing, 1993), 66.

15. Ibid, 149–155.

16. Mark Kastner and Hugh Burroughs. *Alternative Healing: The Complete A to Z Guide to Over 160 Alternative Therapies* (Halcyon Publishing, 1993), 72.

17. Ibid, 93.

18. Ibid, 29.

19. NIH. *Alternative Medicine: Expanding Medical Horizons* (U.S. Government Printing Office, 1993), 183–206.

20. Bill Gottlieb. *New Choices in Natural Healing* (Rodale Press, 1995), 115.

21. Mark Kastner and Hugh Burroughs. *Alternative Healing: The Complete A to Z Guide to Over 160 Alternative Therapies* (Halcyon Publishing, 1993), 127.

22. Burton Goldberg. *Alternative Medicine: The Definitive Guide* (Future Medicine Publishing, 1993), 339–345.

23. NIH. *Alternative Medicine: Expanding Medical Horizons* (U.S. Government Printing Office, 1993), 230–232.

24. Ibid, 222–226.

25. Mark Kastner and Hugh Burroughs. *Alternative Healing: The Complete A to Z Guide to Over 160 Alternative Therapies* (Halcyon Publishing, 1993), 176–178.

26. Ibid, 181.

27. Ibid, 190–192.

28. Doug Podolsky. "A New Age of Healing Hands," U.S. *News & World Report*, February 5, 1996, 74.

29. Bill Gottlieb. *New Choices in Natural Healing* (Rodale Press, 1995), 108–112; Mark Kastner and Hugh Burroughs. *Alternative Healing* (Halcyon Publishing, 1993), 210.

30. Mark Kastner and Hugh Burroughs. *Alternative Healing: The Complete A to Z Guide to Over 160 Alternative Therapies* (Halcyon Publishing, 1993), 232.

31. NIH. *Alternative Medicine: Expanding Medical Horizons* (U.S. Government Printing Office, 1993), 28.

32. Burton Goldberg. *Alternative Medicine: The Definitive Guide* (Future Medicine Publishing, 1993), 422–431; Mark Kastner and Hugh Burroughs. *Alternative Healing* (Halcyon Publishing, 1993), 245.

33. D. Krieger. *Therapeutic Touch: How to Use Your Hands to Help or Heal* (Prentice-Hall, 1979), 34.

CHAPTER SIX: THE M.D. AS AN ALTERNATIVE PRACTITIONER

1. William Collinge. *The American Holistic Health Association Complete Guide to Alternative Medicine* (Warner Books, 1996), 314.

2. George Howe Colt. "See Me, Feel Me, Touch Me, Heal Me," *Life*, September 1996, 36.

3. "Resolution 514 — Alternative (Complementary) Medicine," Reference Committee E, 10–11. From Washington Delegation to American Medical Association House of Delegates.

4. "Alternative Medical Courses Taught at U.S. Medical Schools," The Richard and Hinda Rosenthal Center for Alternative/ Complementary Medicine.

5. Dean Ornish, M.D. *Dr. Dean Ornish's Program for Reversing Hearth Disease* (Ivy Books, 1996).

6. NIH. *Alternative Medicine: Expanding Medical Horizons* (U.S. Government Printing Office, 1993), xli.

7. American Holistic Medical Association brochure.

8. David Eisenberg, M.D. "Unconventional Medicine in the United States," *New England Journal of Medicine*, January 28, 1993, 246.

9. Butch Levy, M.D., L.Ac. Personal interview, June 1996.

10. Ibid.

11. Ibid.

12. Robert Duggan, M.Ac., Dipl.Ac. (NCCA), Personal interview, July 1996.

13. American Holistic Medical Association brochure.

14. Evarts Loomis, M.D., F.A.C.S.I. Personal interview, Fall 1991.

15. Evarts Loomis, M.D., F.A.C.S.I. Personal correspondence, July 1996.

16. Larry Dossey, M.D. Personal interview, Fall 1989.

17. Doug Podlosky. "A New Age of Healing Hands," U.S. *News & World Report*, February 5, 1996, 71–74.

18. American Holistic Medical Association brochure.

19. Butch Levy, M.D., L.Ac. Personal interview, June 1996.

20. Leonard Wisneski, M.D. Personal interview, September 1989.

21. Butch Levy, M.D., L.Ac. Personal interview, June 1996.

22. Ibid.

23. Ibid.

24. Bill Gottlieb. *New Choices in Natural Healing* (Rodale Press, 1995), 68.

25. Mary Walker. "Choosing a Holistic M.D.," East/West Journal, April 1990, 24.

26. Ibid.

27. Butch Levy, M.D., L.Ac. Personal interview, June 1996.

28. Ibid.

29. Ibid.

30. Mary Walker. "Choosing a Holistic M.D.," East/West Journal, April 1990, 211.

31. American Holistic Medical Association brochure.

32. Ibid.

CHAPTER SEVEN: TRADITIONAL CHINESE MEDICINE

1. Burton Goldberg. Alternative Medicine: The Definitive Guide (Future Medicine Publishing, 1993), 450.

2. American Association of Oriental Medicine (AAOM) Fact Sheet.

3. Ibid.

4. Ibid.

5. Ibid.

6. "NIH/PHS Awards in Alternative Medicine," Office of Alternative Medicine (OAM) National Institutes of Health (NIH) Research Information Package.

7. American Association of Oriental Medicine (AAOM) Fact Sheet.

8. Ibid.

9. NIH. Alternative Medicine: Expanding Medical Horizons (U.S. Government Printing Office, 1993), 76.

10. American Association of Oriental Medicine (AAOM) Fact Sheet.

11. Harriet Beinfield, L.Ac. and Effrem Korngold, L.Ac., O.M.D. "Chinese Traditional Medicine: An Introductory Overview," Alternative Therapies in Health and Medicine, March 1995, 45.

12. Ibid.

13. Mary Walker. "Choosing an Acupuncturist," *East/West Journal*, April 1991, 110.

14. Mark Kastner and Hugh Burroughs. *Alternative Healing* (Halcyon Publishing, 1993), 3.

15. Harriet Beinfield, L.Ac., and Effrem Korngold, L.Ac., O.M.D. "Chinese Traditional Medicine: An Introductory Overview," *Alternative Therapies in Health and Medicine*, March 1995, 44.

16. R.H. Bannerman, M.D. The World Health Organization View point on Acupuncture. "WHO Interregional Seminar on Acupuncture, Moxibustion, and Acupuncture Anesthesia," Peking, June 1979.

17. NIH. *Alternative Medicine: Expanding Medical Horizons* (U.S. Government Printing Office, 1993), 72.

18. Gabrielle K. McDonald, U.S. District Court Judge, Houston, TX. Quoted in Mary Walker. "Choosing an Acupuncturist," *East/West Journal*, April 1991, 108.

19. R.H. Bannerman, M.D. The World Health Organization View point on Acupuncture. "WHO Interregional Seminar on Acupuncture, Moxibustion, and Acupuncture Anesthesia," Peking, June 1979.

20. *National Acupuncture Detoxification Association Newsletter* (NADA), December 1992, 1–6.

21. Claudia Wallis. "Why New Age Medicine Is Catching On," *Time*, November 4, 1991, 70.

22. William Collinge. *The American Holistic Health Association Complete Guide to Alternative Medicine* (Warner Books, 1996), 296.

23. Harriet Beinfield, L.Ac. and Effrem Korngold, L.Ac., O.M.D. "Chinese Traditional Medicine: An Introductory Overview," *Alternative Therapies in Health and Medicine*, March 1995, 51.

24. Mark Kastner and Hugh Burroughs. *Alternative Healing: The Complete A to Z Guide to Over 160 Alternative Therapies* (Halcyon Publishing, 1993), 5.

25. NIH. *Alternative Medicine: Expanding Medical Horizons* (U.S. Government Printing Office, 1993), 72.

26. William Collinge. *The American Holistic Health Association Complete Guide to Alternative Medicine* (Warner Books, 1996), 32.

27. Mark Kastner and Hugh Burroughs. *Alternative Healing: The Complete A to Z Guide to Over 160 Alternative Therapies* (Halcyon Publishing, 1993), 202.

28. William Collinge. *The American Holistic Health Association Complete Guide to Alternative Medicine* (Warner Books, 1996), 43.

29. Ted Kaptchuk. Personal interview, Fall 1989.

30. Robert M. Duggan, M.Ac., Dipl.Ac (NCCA). Personal interview, Fall 1989.

31. Ibid.

32. Gail Ludwig. Personal Interview, Winter 1991.

33. Dr. Miki Shima. Personal interview, Fall 1991.

34. Robert M. Duggan, M.Ac., Dipl.Ac (NCCA). Personal interview, Fall 1989.

35. Dr. Miki Shima. Personal interview, Fall 1989.

36. Ted Kaptchuk. Personal interview, Fall 1989.

37. James Collins, CAA staff, "Letter to the Editor" *East-West Journal* — copy to author, July 24, 1991.

CHAPTER EIGHT: NATUROPATHIC MEDICINE

1. Senator Claiborne Pell. Personal letter to Mrs. Hillary Rodham Clinton, March 31, 1993.

2. Burton Goldberg. *Alternative Medicine: The Definitive Guide* (Future Medicine Publishing, 1993), 360.

3. Bastyr University press release, October 4, 1994.

4. "Naturopathic and Major Medical Schools, Comparative Curricula." Document from the American Association of Naturopathic Physicians.

5. "Twenty Questions About Naturopathic Medicine." Document from the American Association of Naturopathic Medicine.

6. "Naturopathic and Major Medical Schools: Comparative Curricula." Document from the American Association of Naturopathic Physicians.

7. William Collinge. *The American Holistic Health Association Complete Guide to Alternative Medicine* (Warner Books, 1996), 125.

8. NIH. *Alternative Medicine: Expanding Medical Horizons* (U.S. Government Printing Office, 1993), 88.

9. American Association of Naturopathic Physicians brochure.

10. Ibid.

11. Bastyr University press release, February 27, 1995.

12. American Association of Naturopathic Physicians brochure.

13. Stephen Speidel, N.D. Personal interview, Summer 1990.

14. Jared Zeff, N.D., L.Ac., Personal interview, June 1996.

15. Ibid.

16. NIH. *Alternative Medicine: Expanding Medical Horizons* (U.S. Government Printing Office, 1993), 89.

17. Dean Ornish, M.D. *Dr. Dean Ornish's Program for Reversing Heart Disease* (Ivy Books, 1996).

18. Konrad Kail, N.D. Personal interview, Fall 1990.

19. Jared Zeff, N.D., L.Ac. Personal interview, June 1996.

20. "NIH Exploratory Study Coordination Centers for Alternative Medical Research." NIH Office of Alternative Medicine press release, June 1995.

21. Jared Zeff, N.D., L.Ac. Personal interview, June 1996.

22. Jim Massey, N.D. Personal interview, August 1990.

23. Yvonne Sklar. Personal correspondence, July 1996.

24. Jared Zeff, N.D., L.Ac. Personal interview, June 1996.

25. Konrad Kail, N.D. Personal interview, Fall 1990.

26. Ibid.

27. American Association of Naturopathic Physicians brochure.

28. Jared Zeff, N.D., L.Ac. Personal interview, June 1996.

29. Jim Massey, N.D. Personal interview, Summer 1990.

CHAPTER NINE: CHIROPRACTIC MEDICINE

1. William Collinge. *The American Holistic Health Association Complete Guide to Alternative Medicine* (Warner Books, 1996), 232.

2. NIH. *Alternative Medicine: Expanding Medical Horizons* (U.S. Government Printing Office, 1993), 121.

3. Brad M. Hayes, D.C. Strategies for Integrating Chiropractic into Managed Care Setting. Presentation at "Integrating Managed Care & Alternative Medicine," San Francisco, CA, December 1995.

4. Ibid.

5. "Mediclaim," State Farm Insurance Companies, November 1992, 6.

6. NIH. *Alternative Medicine: Expanding Medical Horizons* (U.S. Government Printing Office, 1993), 121.

7. Brian Inglis. *History of Medicine* (Weisenfeld & Nicolson, 1965), p. 137.

8. NIH. *Alternative Medicine: Expanding Medical Horizons* (U.S. Government Printing Office, 1993), 120.

9. Stuart Garber, D.C., D. Hom. (MED.) Personal Interview, December 1989.

10. Stuart Garber, D.C., D. Hom. (MED.) Personal correspondence, July 1996.

11. Mary Walker. "Choosing a Chiropractor," *East/West Journal*, February 1991, 28.

12. Ibid.

13. Bernard Jensen, D.C., Ph.D. Personal interview, June 1991.

14. Burton Goldberg. *Alternative Medicine: The Definitive Guide* (Future Medicine Publishing, 1993), 139.

15. P.G. Shekelle et al. "The Appropriateness of Spinal Manipulation for Low-Back Pain: Indications and Ratings by a Multidisciplinary Expert Panel." Rand/UCLA, 1991, Monograph No. R-4025/2-CCR/FCER.

16. R. Smith. "Where Is the Wisdom? The Poverty of Medical Evidence," *British Medical Journal*, October 1991, Vol. 303, 789–799.

17. William Collinge. *The American Holistic Health Association Complete Guide to Alternative Medicine* (Warner Books, 1996), 248.

18. William Collinge. *The American Holistic Health Association Complete Guide to Alternative Medicine* (Warner Books, 1996), 249; P. Brennan, K. Kokjohn, and C. Kaltinger. "Enhanced phagocytic cell respiratory burst induced by spinal manipulation: potential role of substance," *Journal of Manipulative Therapeutics*, 14(7):399–408, 1991.

19. "Government and Research Studies on Chiropractic," National Board of Chiropractic Examiners Brochure.

20. Stuart Garber, D.C., D. Hom. (MED.) Personal interview, December 1989.

21. Fred Lerner, D.C., Ph.D., F.A.C.O. Personal interview, Fall 1989.

22. Ibid.

23. Ibid.

24. Stuart Garber, D.C., D. Hom. (MED.) Personal interview, Fall 1989.

25. Ibid.

26. The Council on Chiropractic Education brochure.

CHAPTER TEN: OSTEOPATHIC MEDICINE

1. American Osteopathic Association brochure.

2. Ibid.

3. William Collinge. *The American Holistic Health Association Complete Guide to Alternative Medicine* (Warner Books, 1996), 207.

4. American Osteopathic Association brochure.

5. Burton Goldberg. *Alternative Medicine: The Definitive Guide* (Future Medicine Publishing, 1993), 410.

6. Harold Magoun, Jr., D.O., F.A.A.O. Personal interview, June 1996.

7. Diane Krstulovich. "When Structure Equals Function," *Vegetarian Times*, June 1994, 91.

8. Obituary for Charles H. Spencer, *Forum of Osteopathy*, March 1940.

9. Diane Krstulovich. "When Structure Equals Function," *Vegetarian Times*, June 1994, 91.

10. Ibid.

11. NIH. *Alternative Medicine: Expanding Medical Horizons* (U.S. Government Printing Office, 1993), 114.

12. I.M. Korr, Ph.D. Personal correspondence, July 1996.

13. Jan Hendryx, D.O. Personal interview, June 1996.

14. I.M. Korr, Ph.D. Personal correspondence, July 1996.

15. Jan Hendryx, D.O. Personal interview, June 1996.

16. I.M. Korr, Ph.D. Personal correspondence, July 1996.

17. Jan Hendryx, D.O. Personal interview, June 1996.

18. Harold Magoun, Jr., D.O., F.A.A.O. Personal correspondence, July 1996.

19. Diane Krstulovich. "When Structure Equals Function," *Vegetarian Times*, June 1994, 90.

20. Dr. Charles Spencer. Personal communication with his wife, Mildred Spencer, 1985.

21. Diane Krstulovich. "When Structure Equals Function," *Vegetarian Times*, June 1994, 90; Harold Magoun, Jr., D.O., F.A.A.O. Personal interview, June 1996.

22. Diane Krstulovich. "When Structure Equals Function," *Vegetarian Times*, June 1994, 90.

23. Harold Magoun, Jr., D.O. Personal interview, June 1996.

24. William Collinge. *The American Holistic Health Association Complete Guide to Alternative Medicine* (Warner Books, 1996), 215.

25. Ibid.

26. Harold Magoun, Jr., D.O. Personal interview, June 1996.

27. Andrew Weil. *Health and Healing* (Houghton Mifflin, 1983), 133.

28. Burton Goldberg. *Alternative Medicine: The Definitive Guide* (Future Medicine Publishing, 1993), 406.

29. Sarah Pattee. "A Touch Opens Door to Healing," *Los Angeles Times*, October 3, 1990.

30. Jan Hendryx, D.O. Personal interview, June 1996.

31. Charles H. Spencer, D.O. "Sane Health Principles," *The Western Osteopath*, July/August 1932, 8.

32. Dr. Charles Spencer. Personal communication with his wife, Mildred Spencer, 1985.

33. Burton Goldberg. *Alternative Medicine: The Definitive Guide* (Future Medicine Publishing, 1993), 406–409; Diane Krstulovich. "When Structure Equals Function," *Vegetarian Times*, June 1994, 91.

34. William Collinge. *The American Holistic Health Association Complete Guide to Alternative Medicine* (Warner Books, 1996), 223.

35. Burton Goldberg. *Alternative Medicine: The Definitive Guide* (Future Medicine Publishing, 1993), 406–407; William Collinge. *The American Holistic Health Association Complete Guide to Alternative Medicine* (Warner Books, 1996), 217–226.

36. William Collinge. *The American Holistic Health Association Complete Guide to Alternative Medicine* (Warner Books, 1996), 225.

37. Susan Rubinstein. "The Osteopathic Alternative," *East/West Journal*, December 1990, 48.

38. Harold Magoun, Jr., D.O. Personal interview, June 1996.

39. "What Makes a D.O. Different?" American Osteopathic Association document.

40. Susan Rubinstein. "The Osteopathic Alternative," *East/West Journal*, December 1990, 46.

41. Harold Magoun, Jr., D.O. Personal correspondence, July 1996.

42. Susan Rubinstein. "The Osteopathic Alternative," *East/West Journal*, December 1990, 47.

ORGANIZATIONS, SUPPORT GROUPS, AND TREATMENT PROGRAMS

- ALTERNATIVE MEDICAL TREATMENT PROGRAMS
- ALTERNATIVE MEDICAL TREATMENT PROGRAMS, SUPPORT GROUPS, and ADVOCACY ORGANIZATIONS
- PROFESSIONAL ORGANIZATIONS and TRADE ASSOCIATIONS
- ALTERNATIVE MEDICAL SCHOOLS and TRAINING PROGRAMS

ACUPRESSURE

Acupressure Institute
1533 Shattuck Ave., Berkeley, CA 94709, 510-845-1059

American Oriental Bodywork Therapy Association
Glenndale Executive Campus, #510, 1000 Whitehorse Rd.
Boorhees, NJ 08043, 609-782-1616

ACUPUNCTURE/TRADITIONAL CHINESE MEDICINE

American Academy of Medical Acupuncture
5820 Wilshire Blvd., Suite 500, Los Angeles, CA 90036
213-937-5514

American Association of Oriental Medicine
433 Front St., Catasaqua, PA 18032, 610-433-2448

Council of Colleges of Acupuncture and Oriental Medicine
1010 Wayne Ave., Suite 1270, Silver Spring, MD 20910
301-608-9175

National Acupuncture and Oriental Medical Alliance
14637 Starr Rd. SE, Olalla, WA 98359, 206-851-6896

National Acupuncture Detoxification Association
P.O. Box 1927, Vancouver, WA 98668, 360-260-8620

National Commission for the Certification of Acupuncturists
1424 16th St. NW, Suite 601, Washington, D.C. 20036
202-232-1404

Traditional Acupuncture Institute
American City Building
10227 Wincopin Circle, Suite 100, Columbia, MD 21044
301-596-6006

ADDICTIONS

National Acupuncture Detoxification Association
349 E. 140th St., Bronx, NY 718-993-3100

Sitike Counseling Center
1211 Mission Rd., South San Francisco, CA 94080, 415-589-9305

AIDS

AIDS ALTERNATIVE HEALTH PROJECT
4753 N. Broadway, Chicago, IL 60640, 312-561-2800

HEAL
16 E. 16th St., New York, NY 10003, 212-674-HOPE

ALLERGIES

American Academy of Environmental Medicine
4510 W. 89th St., Suite 110, Prairie Village, KS 66207, 913-642-6062

ALTERNATIVE MEDICINE

American Foundation for Alternative Health Care
25 Landfield Ave., Monticello, NY 12701, 914-794-8181

The Fetzer Institute
9292 W. KL Ave., Kalamazoo, MI 49009, 616-375-2000

Office of Alternative Medicine (OAM)
National Institutes of Health (NIH)
6120 Executive Blvd., EPS Suite 450, Rockville, MD 20892
301-402-2466.

Richard and Hinda Rosenthal Center for Alternative/
Complementary Medicine
College of Physicians and Surgeons
at Columbia University
630 W. 168th St., New York, NY 10032, 212-305-4755

ALZHEIMER'S DISEASE

Alzheimer's Association
919 N. Michigan Ave., Suite 1000, Chicago, IL 60611, 800-272-3900

AROMATHERAPY

Aromatherapy Institute of Research
P.O. Box 2354, Fair Oaks, CA 95628, 916-965-7546

Aromatherapy Seminars
1830 S. Robertson Blvd., #203, Los Angeles, CA 90035
800-677-2368

National Association for Holistic Aromatherapy
P.O. Box 17622, Boulder, CO 80308, 800-566-6735

The Pacific Institute of Aromatherapy
P.O. Box 6842, San Rafael, CA 94903, 415-479-9121

ART THERAPY

American Art Therapy Association
1202 Allanson Rd., Mundelein, IL 60060, 847-949-6064

AYURVEDIC MEDICINE

American Institute of Ayurvedic Sciences
2115 112th Ave. NE, Bellevue, WA 98004, 206-453-8022

Ayurvedic Institute
P.O.Box 23455, Albuquerque, NM 87192, 505-291-9698

The College of Ayur-Veda Health Center
P.O. Box 282, Fairfield, Iowa 52556, 515-472-8477

BEE VENOM THERAPY (APITHERPY)

American Apitherapy Society
Box 54, Hartland Four Corners, VT 05049, 804-436-2708

BEHAVIORAL (MIND-BODY) MEDICINE

The Center for Mind-Body Studies
5225 Connecticut Ave. NW, Suite 414, Washington, DC, 20015
202-966-7338

Mind-Body Institute
Mercy Hospital and Medical Center, 2525 S. Michigan Ave.
Chicago, IL 60616, 312-567-2259

The Mind-Body Medical Center
Deaconess Hospital, Deaconess Rd., Boston, MA 02215
617-632-9525

The Society of Behavioral Medicine
410 E. Jefferson, Suite 205, Rockville, MD 20850, 301-251-2790

BIOFEEDBACK

Association for Applied Psychophysiology and Biofeedback
10200 W. 44th Ave., Suite 304, Wheatridge, CO 80033
303-422-8436

Center for Applied Psychophysiology
Menninger Clinic, P.O. Box 829, Topeka, KS 66601
913-273-7500, Ext. 5375

BODYWORK/MASSAGE

American Center for the Alexander Technique
129 W. 67th St., New York, NY 10023, 212-799-0468

American Massage Therapy Association
820 Davis St., Suite 100, Evanston, IL 60201, 847-864-0123

Associated Bodywork and Massage Professionals
28677 Buffalo Park Rd., Evergreen, CO 80439, 800-458-2267

The Body of Knowledge/Hellerwork
406 Berry St., Mt. Shasta, CA 96067, 916-926-2500

Bonnie Prudden Myotherapy
3661 N. Campbell Ave., Tucson, AZ 85719, 602-529-3979

Feldenkrais Guild
P.O. Box 489, Albany, OR 97321, 503-926-0981

Guild for Structural Integration
1800 30th, Suite 310, Boulder, CO 80401, 303-447-0122

International Rolf Institute
P.O. Box 1868, Boulder, CO 80306, 303-449-5903

North American Society of Teachers of the Alexander Technique
P.O. Box 3992, Champaign, IL 61826, 800-473-0620

Polarity Wellness Center
132 E. 85th St., #2-1, New York, NY 10028, 212-327-4050

Trager Institute
21 Locust Ave., Mill Valley, CA 94941, 415-388-2688

CANCER

The Arlin J. Brown Information Center
P.O. Box 251, Fort Belvoir, VA 22060, 540-752-9511

Cancer Control Society
2043 North Berendo St., Los Angeles, CA 90027, 213-663-7801

CanHelp
3111 Paradise Bay Rd., Port Ludlow, WA 90365, 360-437-2291

Center for Advancement in Cancer Education
300 E. Lancaster Ave., Wynnewood, PA 19096, 610-642-4810

Commonweal
P.O. Box 316, Bolinas, CA 94924, 415-868-0970

Exceptional Cancer Patients
1302 Chapel St., New Haven, CT 06511, 203-865-8392

Foundation for Advancement in Cancer Therapies
P.O. Box 1242, Old Chelsea Station, New York, NY 10113
212-741-2790

Geffen Cancer Center
981 37th Place, Vero Beach, FL 32960, 800-834-4791

International Association for Cancer Victors and Friends
7740 W. Manchester Ave., Suite 203, Playa del Rey, CA 90293
310-822-5032

National Coalition for Cancer Survivorship
1010 Wayne Ave., Suite 505, Silver Spring, MD 20901
301-650-8868

Patient Advocates for Advanced Cancer Treatments (PAACT)
1143 Parmelee NW, Grand Rapids, MI 49504, 616-453-1477

People Against Cancer
P.O. Box 10, Otho, IA 50569, 515-972-4444

Simonton Cancer Center
P.O. Box 890, Pacific Palisades, CA 90272, 310-457-3811

The Wellness Community
2716 Ocean Park Blvd., Suite 1040, Santa Monica, CA 90403
310-314-2555

Wainwright House
260 Stuyvesant Ave., Rye, NY 10580, 914-967-6080

Windhorse Corporation
3939 Houma Blvd., #4, Bldg #2, Metarie, LA 70006, 504-888-1320

World Research Foundation
15300 Ventura Blvd., Suite 405, Sherman Oaks, CA 91403
818-907-5483

CHELATION THERAPY

American Board of Chelation Therapy
1407-B N. Wells, Chicago, IL 60610, 800-356-2228

American College for Advancement in Medicine
P.O. Box 3427, Laguna Hills, CA 92654, 714-583-7666

The Rheumatoid Disease Foundation
5106 Old Harding Rd., Franklin, TN 37064, 615-646-1030

CHIROPRACTIC MEDICINE

American Chiropractic Association
1701 Clarendon Blvd., Arlington, VA 22209, 703-276-8800

International Chiropractors Association
1100 N. Glebe Rd., Suite 1000, Arlington, VA 22201
703-528-5000

World Chiropractic Alliance
2950 N. Dobson Rd., Suite 1, Chandler, AZ 85224, 800-347-1011

Association for Network Chiropractic Spinal Analysis
P.O. Box 7682, Longmont, CO 80501, 303-678-8101

International Board of Applied Kinesiology
6405 Metcalf Ave., Suite 503, Shawnee Mission, KS 66202
913-384-5336

CHRONIC FATIGUE SYNDROME

CFIDS Association
P.O. Box 220398, Charlotte, NC 28222, 800-442-3437

COLON THERAPY

International Association for Colon-Hydrotherapy
2204 N.W. Loop, Suite 410, San Antonio, TX 78230, 210-366-2888

Wood Hygienic Institute
P.O. Box 420580, Kissimmee, FL 34742, 407-933-0009

CRANIALSACRAL THERAPY

The Cranial Academy
3500 Depaw Blvd., Indianapolis, IN 46286, 317-594-0411

SORSI (Sacral Occipital Technique)
P.O. Box 8245, Prairie Village, KS 66208, 913-649-3475

The Upledger Institute
11211 Prosperity Farms Rd., Palm Beach Gardens, FL 33410
407-622-4706

DANCE/MOVEMENT THERAPY

American Dance Therapy Association
2000 Century Plaza, Suite 108, Columbia, MD 21044, 410-997-4040

DENTISTRY (HOLISTIC AND BIOLOGICAL)

American Academy of Biological Dentistry
P.O. Box 856, Carmel Valley, CA 93924, 408-659-5385

Environmental Dental Association
9974 Scripps Ranch Blvd., Suite 36, San Diego, CA 92131
800-388-8124

DIET AND NUTRITION

American College of Advancement in Medicine
P.O. Box 3427, Laguna Hills, CA 92654, 714-583-7666

Kushi Institute
P.O. Box 7, Becket, MA 01223, 413-623-5741

ENERGY MEDICINE/SUBTLE ENERGY

American Polarity Therapy Association
2888 Bluff St., Suite 149, Boulder, CO 80301, 303-545-2080

American-International Reiki Association
2210 Wilshire Blvd., Suite 831, Santa Monica, CA 90403

International Society for the Study of Subtle Energies
and Energy Medicine (ISSSEEM)
356 Goldco Circle, Golden, CO 80401, 303-278-2228

Reiki Alliance
P.O. Box 41, Cataldo, ID 83810, 208-682-3535

ENVIRONMENTAL MEDICINE

American Academy of Environmental Medicine
4510 W. 89th St., Suite 110, Prairie Village, KS 66207
913-642-6062

Environmental Health Center
8345 Walnut Hill Lane, Suite 205, Dallas, TX 75231, 214-368-4132

Human Ecology Action League
P.O. Box 29629, Atlanta, GA 30359, 404-248-1898

FLOWER REMEDIES AND ESSENCE THERAPY

Ellon Bach U.S.A.
644 Merrick Rd., Lynbrook, NY 11563, 516-593-2206

The Flower Essence Society
P.O. Box 459, Nevada City, CA 95959, 800-548-0075

GUIDED IMAGERY

Academy of Guided Imagery
P.O. Box 2070, Mill Valley, CA 94942, 800-726-2070

Center for Applied Psychophysiology
Menninger Clinic, P.O. Box 829, Topeka, KS 66601
913-273-7500, Ext. 5375

International Imagery Association
P.O. Box 1046, Bronx, NY 10471, 914-423-9200

HEART DISEASE AND CARDIAC RISK

Heart Disease Reversal Clinic
Duke University Medical Center, 1821 Green St.
Durham, NC 27705, 919-286-2243

Preventive Medicine Research Institute
900 Bridgeway, Suite 2, Sausalito, CA 94965, 415-332-2525

HERBOLOGY

American Association of Naturopathic Physicians
2366 Eastlake Ave. E, Suite 322, Seattle, WA 98102
206-323-7610

American Botanical Council
P.O. Box 201660, Austin, TX 78720, 512-331-8868

American Herbalist Guild
P.O. Box 746555, Arvada, CO 80006, 303-423-8800

Herb Research Foundation
1007 Pearl St., Suite 200, Boulder, CO 80302, 303-449-2265

Institute for Traditional Medicine
2017 S.E. Hawthorne, Portland, OR 97214, 503-233-4907

HOLISTIC MEDICINE AND HOLISTIC HEALTH

American Holistic Health Association
P.O. Box 17400, Anaheim, CA 92817, 714-779-6152

American Holistic Medical Association
4101 Boone Lake Trail, Suite 201, Raleigh, NC 27607, 919-787-5146

American Holistic Nurses Association
4101 Boone Lake Trail, Suite 201, Raleigh, NC 27607, 919-787-5181

Association of Holistic Healing Centers
109 Holly Crescent, Suite 201, Virginia Beach, VA 23451

HOMEOPATHIC MEDICINE

British Institute of Homeopathy and College of Homeopathy
520 Washington Blvd., Suite 423, Marina Del Rey, CA 90292
310-306-5408

Homeopathic Association of Naturopathic Physicians
P.O. Box 12488, Portland, OR 97212, 503-795-0579

Homeopathic Eduational Services
2124 Kittredge St., Berkeley, CA 94704, 510-649-0294

National Center for Homeopathy
801 N. Fairfax St., Suite 306, Alexandria, VA 22314, 703-548-7790

National College of Naturopathic Medicine
11231 S.E. Market St., Portland, OR 97216, 503-255-4860

New England School of Homeopathy
115 Elm St., Suite 210, Enfield, CT 06082, 800-637-4440

HOSPICE, DEATH AND DYING

National Hospice Organization
1901 N. Moore St., Suite 901, Arlington, VA 22209, 703-243-5900

HUMOR THERAPY

American Association for Therapeutic Humor
222 S. Meramec, Suite 303, St. Louis, MO 63105, 314-863-6232

HYDROTHERAPY

Uchee Pines Institute
30 Uchee Pines Rd., Suite 75, Seale, AL 36975, 334-855-4781

HYPNOTHERAPY

The American Institute of Hypnotherapy
16842 Von Karman, Suite 475, Irvine, CA 92714, 714-261-640

The American Society of Clinical Hypnosis
2200 E. Devon Ave., Suite 91, Des Plaines, IL 60018
847-297-3317

INFORMED CHOICE/PATIENT INFORMATION

American Self-Help Clearinghouse
Northwest Covenant Medical Center, 25 Pocano Rd.
Denville, NJ 07834, 201-625-7101

Archaeus Project
P.O. Box 7079, Kamuela, HI 96743, 808-885-6773

Committee for Freedom of Choice in Medicine
1180 Walnut Ave., Chula Vista, CA 91911, 800-227-4473

Office of Alternative Medicine (OAM),
National Institutes of Health
6120 Executive Blvd., EPS Suite 450, Rockville, MD 20892
301-402-2466

The Picker Institute
1295 Boylston St., Suite 100, Boston, MA 02215, 617-667-2388

Planetree Health Resource Center
2040 Webster, San Francisco, CA 94115, 415-923-3681

Price-Pottenger Nutrition Foundation
P.O. Box 2614, La Mesa, CA 91943, 800-366-3748

Rise Institute
P.O. Box 2733, Petaluma, CA 94973, 707-765-2758

IRIDOLOGY

Bernard Jensen International
24360 Old Wagon Wheel Rd., Escondido, CA 92027, 619-749-2727

National Iridology Research Association
1101 W. Main, Suite R, League City, TX 77573, 713-554-2626

LIGHT THERAPY AND COLOR THERAPY

College of Syntonic Optometry
1200 Robeson St., Fall River, MA 02720, 508-673-1251

Dinshaw Health Society
P.O. Box 707, Malaga, NJ 08328, 609-692-4686

Environmental Health & Light Research Institute
3923 Coconut Palm Dr., Suite 101, Tampa, FL 33619, 800-544-4878

MAGNETIC FIELD THERAPY

Bio-Electro-Magnetics Institute
2490 W. Moana Lane, Reno, NV 89509, 702-827-9099

International Society for the Study of Subtle Energy
& Energy Medicine
356 Goldco Circle, Golden, CO 80403, 303-278-1228

MEDITATION/RELAXATION TECHNIQUES

Center for Spiritual Awareness
P.O. Box 7, Lake Rabun Rd., Lakemont, GA 30552, 706-782-4723

Institute for Noetic Sciences
P.O. Box 909, Sausalito, CA 94966, 415-331-5650

Maharishi International University
1000 N. 4th St., Fairfield, IA 52557, 515-472-7000

The Mind-Body Medical Institute
Deaconess Hospital, Deaconess Rd., Boston, MA 02215
617-632-9525

MIDWIFERY

American College of Nurse-Midwives
818 Connecticut Ave. NW, Suite 900, Washington, DC 20006
202-728-9860

NATUROPATHIC MEDICINE

American Association of Naturopathic Physicians
2366 Eastlake Ave. E, Suite 322, Seattle, WA 98102
206-323-7610

Bastyr University of Natural Health Sciences
144 N.E. 54th St., Seattle, WA 98105, 206-523-9585

National College of Naturopathic Medicine
11231 S.E. Market St., Portland, OR 97216, 503-255-4860

Southwest College of Naturopathic Medicine & Health Sciences
6535 E. Osborn Rd., Scottsdale, AZ 85251, 602-990-7424

The Canadian College of Naturopathic Medicine
2300 Jonge St., 18th Floor, Box 2431, Toronto, Ontario, Canada
M4PIE4, 416-486-8584

ORTHOMOLECULAR MEDICINE/ VITAMIN AND MINERAL THERAPY

American College for Advancement in Medicine
P.O. Box 3427, Laguna Hills, CA 92654, 714-583-7666

Linus Pauling Institute of Science and Medicine
440 Page Mill Rd., Palo Alto, CA 94306, 415-327-4064

Price-Pottenger Nutrition Foundation
P.O. Box 2614, La Mesa, CA 91943, 800-366-3748

OSTEOPATHIC MEDICINE

American Academy of Osteopathy
3500 DePauw Blvd., Suite 1080, Indianapolis, IN 46268
317-879-1881

American Osteopathic Association
142 E. Ontario St., Chicago, IL 60611, 312-280-5800

OXYGEN (OZONE) THERAPY

The American College of Hyperbaric Medicine
Ocean Medical Center, 4001 Ocean Dr., Suite 105
Lauderdale-by-the-Sea, FL 33308, 305-771-4000

International Association for Oxygen Therapy
P.O. Box 1360, Priest River, IA 83856, 208-448-2504

International Bio-oxidative Medicine Foundation
P.O. Box 891954, Oklahoma City, OK 73189, 405-478-IBOM

International Ozone Association
31 Strawberry Hill Ave., Stamford, CT 06902, 203-348-3542

PAIN

The American Academy of Neural Therapy
1468 S. Saint France Drive, Santa Fe, NM 87501, 505-988-308

American Chronic Pain Association
P.O. Box 850, Rocklin, CA 95677, 916-632-0922

Shealy Institute for Comprehensive Pain and Health Center
1328 E. Evergreen, Springfield, MO 65803, 417-865-5940

St. John Neuromuscular Pain Relief Institute
10710 Seminole Blvd., Suite 2, Seminole, FL 34648, 813-392-2699

PREVENTIVE MEDICINE

American Preventive Medical Association
459 Walker Rd., Great Falls, VA 22066, 800-230-2762

REFLEXOLOGY

American Reflexology Certification Board
P.O. Box 620607, Littleton, CO 80162, 303-933-6921

Foot Reflexology Awareness Association
P.O. Box 7622, Mission Hills, CA 91346, 818-361-0528

International Institute of Reflexology
P.O. Box 12642, St. Petersburg, FL 33733, 813-343-4811

Reflexology Center
41 Park Ave., Suite 8A, New York, NY 10016, 800-FEET-FIRST

SOUND AND MUSIC THERAPY

American Association for Music Therapy
1 Station Plaza, Ossining, NY 10562, 914-944-9260

The Chalice of Repose Project
St. Patricks Hospital, 554 W. Broadway, Missoula, MT 59802
406-542-0001, Ext. 2810

The Institute for Music, Health, and Education
3010 Hennepin Ave., Minneapolis, MN 55408, 612-377-5700

National Association for Music Therapy
8455 Colesville Rd., Suite 930, Silver Springs, MD 20910
301-589-3300

Sound and Listening Center
2701 E. Camelback, Suite 205, Phoenix, AZ 85016, 602-381-0086

STRESS

The Stress Reduction Clinic, Department of Medicine
University of Massachusetts Medical Center, Worcester, MA 01655
508-856-2656

T'AI CHI/ QIGONG

American Foundation of Tradition Chinese Medicine
505 Beach St., San Francisco, CA 94133, 415-776-0502

The Healing Tao Center
P.O. Box 1194, Huntington, NY 11743, 516-367-2701

Qigong Institute/East-West Academy of Healing Arts
450 Sutter St., Suite 916, San Francisco, CA 94108, 415-788-2227

THERAPEUTIC TOUCH

National League for Nursing
350 Hudson St., New York, NY 10014, 800-669-9656

Nurse Healers Professional Association
P.O. Box 444, Allison Park, PA 15101, 412-355-8476

WELLNESS

The National Wellness Association
1045 Clark St., Suite 210, Stevens Point, WI 54881, 715-342-2969

WOMAN'S HEALTH

National Women's Health Network
514 10th St. NW, Suite 400, Washington, D.C. 20004, 202-347-1140

Women to Women
One Pleasant St., Yarmouth, ME 04096, 207-846-6163

YOGA

American Yoga Association
513 South Orange Ave., Sarasota, FL 34236, 800-226-5859

Himalayan International Institute
RR #1, Box 400, Honesdale, PA 18431, 800-822-4547

International Association of Yoga Therapists
109 Hillside Ave., Mill Valley, CA 94941, 415-381-0876

Rocky Mountain Institute of Yoga and Ayurveda
P.O. Box 1091, Boulder, CO 80306, 303-443-6923

MEDICAL AND HEALTH INFORMATION SERVICE ORGANIZATIONS

CANHELP
3111 Paradise Bay Road, Port Ludlow, WA 98365, 360-437-2291

Specializes in reliable information about cancer and cancer treatments, including unconventional and alternative treatments, as well as specialists and treatment centers.

The Health Resource, Inc.
Locust Avenue, Conway, AR 72032, 800-949-0090

Includes alternative medical treatment options and information from international databases. Cost $195 ($295 for cancer). A medical update is available for $95 one year after the initial report.

HERMES Consumer Medical Searches
269 Reservation Road, P.O. Box 111, Marina, CA 93933
800-484-9863, ext #5773

Reports of journal articles, medical abstracts, newspaper clips, as well as lists of practitioners for some conditions. Cost $49.50 (three excerpts), $89.95 (10 excerpts) $179.50 (19 excerpts).

Medical Information Service
3000 Sand Hill Road, Bldg #2, Suite 260, Menlo Park, CA 94025
800-999-1999

Journals and articles. Prices start at $89.95 and up depending on how extensive a search.

Planetree Health Resource Center
2040 Webster St. San Francisco, CA 94115, 415-923-3681

> Comprehensive search including copies of relevant articles. Extensive alternative medical treatment information available. Cost $100.

Schine On-Line Services
39 Brenton Avenue, Providence, RI 02906, 800-346-3287

> Cost $100, (Cancer: $189). Database searches including clinical trials.

World Research Foundation
15300 Ventura Blvd, Suite 405, Sherman Oaks, CA 91403
818-907-5483

> Extensive database information available with formatted reports on a number of health conditions. Extensive alternative medical information. Cost $67.50.

ALTERNATIVE MEDICINE INTERNET RESOURCES

WORLD WIDE WEB SITES

The following can serve as jumping off points for a vast array of alternative/unconventional medical and health care information and resources, including databases.

Alternative Medicine Homepage
http://www.pitt.edu/~cbw/altm.html

Alternative Medicine
http://www-hsl.mcmaster.ca/tomflem/altmed.html

Dr. Bowers Complementary and Alternative Medicine Home Page
http://galen.med.virginia.edu/~pj3bs/ComplementaryHome-
Page.html

Health World Online
http://www.healthy.net

Healthcare Publications for Consumers
http://www.ihr.com/publcons.html

Holistic Internet Resources
http://www.hir.com/

Internet and On-Line Resources (Alternative Medicine)
http://www.Halcyon.com/Libastyr/netbib.html

MedWeb: Alternative Medicine
http://www.Gen.Emory.edu/medweb/medweb.altmed.html

Yahoo Health: Alternative Medicine
http://www.yahoo.com/Health/Alternative_Medicine/

U.S. MEDICAL SCHOOLS OFFERING COURSES IN ALTERNATIVE MEDICINE

PROVIDED BY
THE RICHARD AND HINDA ROSENTHAL CENTER FOR
ALTERNATIVE/COMPLEMENTARY MEDICINE

Albert Einstein College of Medicine
"Complementary Medicine"
718-920-5522

Boston University School of Medicine
"Public Health Perspectives on Alternative Health Care"
617-638-5042

Case Western Reserve University School of Medicine
"Chinese Qigong, I & II"
202-966-7338

City University of New York Medical School
(See Mount Sinai School of Medicine.)

Columbia University College of Physicians and Surgeons
"Survey in Alternative/Complementary Medicine"
"T'ai Chi for Patients and Practitioners"
212-535-1012

Cornell Medical College
"Complementary Medicine"
212-639-8137

Eastern Virginia Medical School
"Complementary & Alternative Medicine"
757-446-7462

Emory University School of Medicine
"Complementary Medical Practices"
404-727-5948

Georgetown University School of Medicine
"The Program of Mind-Body Studies"
202-966-7338

Harvard Medical School
"Alternative Medicine:Implications for Clinical Practice
    and Research"
617-667-3995
"Medical Hypnosis and Behavioral Therapy"
617-728-2991

Howard University College of Medicine
"Alternative Medicine, Preventive Medicine, and Decision Making"
202-337-5855

Indiana University School of Medicine
"Complementary Medicine, Developing New Health Paradigms"
317-274-4662

Jefferson Medical College of Thomas Jefferson University
"Seminar in Alternative/Complementary Medicine"
"Mindfulness Meditation Based Stress Management"
"Spiritual Seminar"
215-955-6844

John Hopkins School of Medicine
"The Philosophy and Practice of Healing"
410-955-7894

Medical College of Pennsylvania
"Folk & Popular Health Care Alternatives I"
"Folk & Popular Health Care Alternatives II"
215-842-6540

Mount Sinai School of Medicine
"Survey Course in Alternative Medicine""
"The Power of Subtle Body: Innovative Qigong"
"Mind-Body Techniques and Healing"
"Hypnotherapy"
"Introduction to Biofeedback Techniques and Medical Practice"
"Preparation for Certification in Biofeedback"
215-955-6844

New York Medical College
"Alternative Therapies with Special Focus on Acupuncture
    and Homeopathy"
914-993-4378

Ohio State University College of Medicine
"Maharishi Ayur-Veda"
614-293-3976

Penn State College of Medicine
"Folk and Alternative Health Systems"
717-531-8037

Southern Illinois University School of Medicine
"Chinese Acupuncture"
217-782-7711
"Comparative Systems of Healing"
217-782-5770

Stanford University School of Medicine
"Alternative Medicine: A Scientific View"
408-885-4146

SUNY at Buffalo School of Medicine
"Alternative/Complementary Modalities"
716-887-8227

Tufts University School of Medicine
"Survey Course in Alternative Medicine"
617-641-1901

Uniformed Services University of the Health Sciences
"Alternative Medicine Seminar Series"
202-782-6418

University of Arizona School of Medicine
"Program in Integrative Medicine"
602-647-7858

University of California, Los Angeles School of Medicine
"Psychoneuroimmunology"
310-825-0249
"Medical Acupuncture for Physicians"
510-841-7600
"Introduction to Complementary Medicine"
818-364-3205
"Integrative East West Medicine"
310-206-1895

University of California, San Francisco School of Medicine
"The Healer's Art"
415-868-2642
"Introduction to Homeopathic Medicine"
707-545-1554
"Complementary Ways of Healing"
415-476-3185

University of Cincinnati School of Medicine
"Alternative Approaches to Medical Treatment"
513-558-4066

University of Louisville School of Medicine
"Alternative and Paranormal Health Claims"
"Behavioral Medicine"
"Alternative Medicine"
502-852-6185
502-852-6287

University of Maryland School of Medicine
"Introduction to Complementary (Alternative) Medicine"
410-328-3780

University of Miami School of Medicine
"Art and Science of Acupuncture"
305-548-4751

University of New Mexico
"Alternative Medicine Course"
505-277-6611

University of North Carolina, Chapel Hill School of Medicine
"Principles and Practices of Alternative &
Complementary Medicine"
919-966-5945

University of Virginia School of Medicine
"Healing Options: Complementary Medicine
for Physicians of the Future"
804-924-2094

University of Washington School of Medicine
"Alternative Approaches to Healing"
206-6116-1817

Wayne State School of Medicine
"Introduction to Alternative/Complementary Medicine"
313-577-1147

Yale School of Medicine
"Alternative Medicine in Historical Perspectives"
203-785-4338
"The Mind and Medicine"
203-624-9411

Index

A

ACKNOWLEDGMENTS

Our deep thanks and appreciation to the following people and organizations whose personal and professional support helped make this book possible:

Alan Adams, D.C.; Eric Andresen; Desirée Avalon; Sloan Bashinsky; Angela Barfield; Dean Bender, D.C.; Julianne Blake; Joan Borysenko, Ph.D.; Susan Bradley; Mrs. Joan Brady; Kai Bravo; Bonnie Brody; Hyla Cass, M.D.; Peter Chocka, N.D.; Mrs. Norman Cousins; Deborah Daly and the Richard and Hinda Rosenthal Center for Alternative/Complementary Medicine, Columbia University; Larry Dossey, M.D.; Barbara Dossey, R.N.; Robert Duggan, M.Ac., Dipl.Ac. (NCCA); Chris Dyer; Peter and Peggy Eggers; David Eisenberg, M.D.; the Evergreen Colorado Branch of the Jefferson County Public Library; Adele Friedman; Laurie Friedman; Astrid Forbes; Stuart Garber, D.C.; Ben and Mary Greig; Jan Guthrie and The Health Resource; Milt Hammerly, M.D.; Richard and Lynn Hansen; Carol Hedgedus and the Fetzer Institute; Jan Hendryx, D.O.; Christine Hibbard, Ph.D.; David Hibbard, M.D.; Mark Hochwinder; Joe Jacobs, M.D.; Bernard Jensen, D.C.; Konrad Kail, N.D.; Ted Kaptchuk, O.M.D.; Irvin Korr, Ph.D.; Stan Krippner, Ph.D.; David Lee; Fred Lerner, D.C.; Joanie Lerner; Butch Levy, M.D., L.Ac.; Evarts Loomis, M.D.; Cindy Palay Lyons, L.Ac.; Peggy McConnell; Peggy McDonnell; Barbara Magers and the A.T. Still Memorial Library; Kirksville College of Osteopathic Medicine; Harold Magoun, Jr., D.O.; Mark Mayell;

Robin Mayfield, D.C.; Gary Miller, Ph.D.; Lynn Morris; James Anthony Morton; Lloyd Ney; Christiane Northrup, M.D.; Terry Olsen; Janet Quinn, R.N., Ph.D.; Dean Raffelock, D.C.; Stephanie Raffelock; Steven and LaVerne Ross and the World Research Foundation; Beverly Rubik, Ph.D.; Harvey and Susan Ruderian; Lisa Salyard-Brussel; Norman Shealy, M.D.; Melanie and Jerry Shennan; Benjamin Shield, Ph.D.; Bernie Siegel, M.D.; Yvonne Sklar; James Strohecker and HealthWorld OnLine; Hal and Llorin Teters; Yogan Totain; John Upledger, D.O.; Virginia Wadsworth; Suzan Walters and the American Holistic Health Association; John Weeks; Charles B. Wessel, M.L.S.; Falk Library of the Health Sciences; University of Pittsburgh; Victoria West; Leonard Wisneski, M.D.; Jared Zeff, N.D.

Special thanks to Marilyn McGuire who encouraged us to do this book, Gina Misiroglu who taught us how to write this book, Brie Stranahan Miller and Mary Stranahan who supported this book, and Becky Benenate and Munro Magruder at New World Library who believed in this book.

About the Authors

Mary Walker Morton's personal experience overcoming scoliosis through unconventional treatment became the basis for a lifelong study of alternative medicine. Today she is a nationally recognized journalist specializing in patients' rights and health care education. Her series of articles in *Natural Health* magazine on choosing alternative medicine provided a comprehensive overview of holistic treatments and is reprinted by major associations, licensing boards, and schools to educate consumers.

A key advisor on alternative medicine, Michael Alan Morton, Ph.D., has more than 25 years of experience in health care management. He is the founding president of the American Holistic Health Association (AHHA), and a past trustee of the American Holistic Medical Association. While a program associate at the Fetzer Institute, he chaired a global conference on health care that brought together over one thousand delegates from twenty-eight countries. He has consulted and advised in a wide range of industries in both the private and nonprofit sectors. The Mortons live in Evergreen, Colorado, with their children Nicholas, John, and Deana.

Please feel free to share thoughts and personal stories with the authors at the following address: Michael Alan Morton / Mary Walker Morton, c/o New World Library, 14 Pamaron Way, Novato, CA 94949. Or e-mail the Mortons at 5steps@healthy.net.

NEW WORLD LIBRARY
is dedicated to publishing books
and cassettes that inspire and challenge us
to improve the quality of our lives and our world.

For a catalog of our fine books
and cassettes contact:

NEW WORLD LIBRARY
14 Pamaron Way
Novato, CA 94949
Phone: (415) 884–2100
FAX: (415) 884–2199

Or call toll free: (800) 227–3900